Ranjit Uppal

Lasers and Their Clinical Applications

Ranjit Uppal

Lasers and Their Clinical Applications

Lasers in Dentistry

LAP LAMBERT Academic Publishing

Impressum/Imprint (nur für Deutschland/only for Germany)
Bibliografische Information der Deutschen Nationalbibliothek: Die Deutsche Nationalbibliothek verzeichnet diese Publikation in der Deutschen Nationalbibliografie; detaillierte bibliografische Daten sind im Internet über http://dnb.d-nb.de abrufbar.
Alle in diesem Buch genannten Marken und Produktnamen unterliegen warenzeichen-, marken- oder patentrechtlichem Schutz bzw. sind Warenzeichen oder eingetragene Warenzeichen der jeweiligen Inhaber. Die Wiedergabe von Marken, Produktnamen, Gebrauchsnamen, Handelsnamen, Warenbezeichnungen u.s.w. in diesem Werk berechtigt auch ohne besondere Kennzeichnung nicht zu der Annahme, dass solche Namen im Sinne der Warenzeichen- und Markenschutzgesetzgebung als frei zu betrachten wären und daher von jedermann benutzt werden dürften.

Coverbild: www.ingimage.com

Verlag: LAP LAMBERT Academic Publishing GmbH & Co. KG
Dudweiler Landstr. 99, 66123 Saarbrücken, Deutschland
Telefon +49 681 3720-310, Telefax +49 681 3720-3109
Email: info@lap-publishing.com

Herstellung in Deutschland:
Schaltungsdienst Lange o.H.G., Berlin
Books on Demand GmbH, Norderstedt
Reha GmbH, Saarbrücken
Amazon Distribution GmbH, Leipzig
ISBN: 978-3-8433-2519-6

Imprint (only for USA, GB)
Bibliographic information published by the Deutsche Nationalbibliothek: The Deutsche Nationalbibliothek lists this publication in the Deutsche Nationalbibliografie; detailed bibliographic data are available in the Internet at http://dnb.d-nb.de.
Any brand names and product names mentioned in this book are subject to trademark, brand or patent protection and are trademarks or registered trademarks of their respective holders. The use of brand names, product names, common names, trade names, product descriptions etc. even without a particular marking in this works is in no way to be construed to mean that such names may be regarded as unrestricted in respect of trademark and brand protection legislation and could thus be used by anyone.

Cover image: www.ingimage.com

Publisher: LAP LAMBERT Academic Publishing GmbH & Co. KG
Dudweiler Landstr. 99, 66123 Saarbrücken, Germany
Phone +49 681 3720-310, Fax +49 681 3720-3109
Email: info@lap-publishing.com

Printed in the U.S.A.
Printed in the U.K. by (see last page)
ISBN: 978-3-8433-2519-6

"Dedicated to my parents and guides"

"ACKNOWLEDGEMENTS"

The beauty of life lies not in the belief that all goes smooth and easy but in the endeavor to have the strength to look in the eye of challenge confidently and fearlessly. I pray to God, who has been more than generous and kind to me to instill these qualities in all of us and make us better medical professionals.

*I thank him for endowing me with a wonderful teacher, **Dr.Ranjan Malhotra**, (Professor & Head, Department of Periodontology and Oral Implantology)who has been very kind. I got an opportunity to learn a lot from him and I shall remain indebted to him forever.*

*I owe my special thanks to **Dr. Deepak Grover** (Assisstant Professor, Director Execution) for his constant encouragement, support and motivation throughout my graduation and post-graduation. He always helped me selflessly and took care of me as an elder brother for which I shall remain indebted to him forever.*

*I owe my deepest gratitude to my supervisor **Dr. Vishakha Grover** & **Dr. V.S Battu** (Professor, Periodontology & Oral Implantology) for their detailed review, constructive criticism and excellent advice. Their ideals and concepts have had a remarkable influence on me. Their extensive discussions around my work and interesting explorations have been very helpful for the completion of this project.*

*I owe my special thanks to my revered teacher and Co-guide **Dr. Jasvinder Singh Narula** (Asso.Professor, Periodontology & Oral Implantology) for his excellent guidance, judicious advice and constant encouragement from commencement to completion of this effort. I truly thank him for his selfless contribution of time and close supervision throughout the project.*

2

I am deeply indebted to **Dr. Anoop Kapoor** *(Asso. Professor, Periodontology & Oral Implantology) and* **Dr Jagjit Singh Dhaliwal** *(Professor, Periodontology & Oral Implantology),* **Dr. Shivani Dhawan** *(Reader, Periodontology & Oral Implantology) for their valuable guidance and advice which has filled a sense of respect and love for them. I am thankful to these teachers for clearing my doubts related to the subject.*

A word of thanks to our president **Col. G.S Sandhu** *for providing such a nice library and web services.*

A special thanks to **Dr. Jasjit Sahota** *and* **Dr. Chahat Singh** *for providing such a nice assistance during this project.*

A word of thanks to **Dr. Supreet Kaur** *(MDS), who directly or indirectly contributed towards this academic effort.*

Dr. Ranjit Singh Uppal

CONTENTS

Sr. No.		Page No.
1.	Introduction	7-8
2.	History	9-16
3.	Laser physics	17
4.	Properties of laser	17-20
5.	Components of typical laser	21-27
6.	Mode of delivery of laser	27-33
7.	Tissue interaction of lasers	33-39
8.0	Types of lasers	39-61
8.1	Soft tissue lasers	40-41
8.2	Hard tissue lasers	41
8.3	Wavelengths of lasers	41-42
8.4	Carbondioxide lasers	43-46
8.5	Argon laser	46-48
8.6	Nd:YAG laser	48-51
8.7	HOL:YAG laser	51-52
8.8	ER:YAG laser	52-55

8.9	Diode laser	56-58
8.10	KTP laser	58-59
8.11.	Q- switched laser	59
8.12	FLPPD laser	59
8.13	Copper Vapor laser	60
8.14	Excimer laser	60
8.15	Alexandrite laser	61
8.16	Advantages of lasers	61-62
8.17	Disadvantages of lasers	62
8.18	Hazards of lasers	63-64
8.19	Preventive measures	65-66
9.0	Clinical applications	67-69
9.1	Laser periotherapy	69
9.2	Non surgical therapy with lasers	70-71
9.3	Surgical laser therapy	72
9.4	De-epithelization	73-75
9.5	Osseous surgery	75-76
9.6	Frenectomy	76
9.7	Gingivectomy/Gingivoplasty	77-78

9.8	Crown lengthening	79
9.9	De-pigmentation	79-80
9.10	Free gingival graft	81
10.	Lasers in Dental Implantology	82-85
11.	Low level laser therapy	86-87
12.	Future applications	88-89
13.	Bibliography	90-97

INTRODUCTION

The word laser conjures in the mind's eye many aspects of what might be described as 'modern' life. The words 'powerful', 'precise' and 'innovative' complement our conception of the world in terms of technology, whereas patients often associate the words 'magical' and 'lightening quick' with the use of lasers in medical practice.

Light has been used as a therapeutic agent for many centuries. From the time when Greek practiced heleiotherapy (that is exposure of the body to sun) for restoration of health to the Chinese phototherapy for the treatment of rickets skin cancer & even psychosis.

Phototherapy or the use of light has played a very important role [53].

"**LASER**, an acronym for light amplification by stimulated emission of Radiation" is a device for generating high intensity ostensibly parallel beam of monochromatic electromagnetic radiation[10]. The possibility of stimulated emission was predicted by **Einstein in 1917**[63] which he explained in his treatise "Zur Quantum Theorie Der Starlung". **Schawlow and Townes in 1958** Einstein's theory of stimulated emission and with advent of Bohr's theory of optical resonators were able to describe the principle of MASER (Microwave Amplification by Stimulated Radiation) [29,31,36,53].

Based on Albert Einstein's theory of spontaneous and stimulated emission of radiation, **Maiman** developed the first laser prototype in 1960. Maiman's device used a crystal medium of ruby that emitted a coherent radiant light from the crystal when stimulated by energy. Thus, the ruby laser was created. Shortly thereafter, in 1961, Snitzer published the prototype for the Nd:YAG laser.

The first application of a laser to dental tissue was reported by **Goldman et al**.; and **Stern and Sognnaes**, in 1964, describing the effects of the ruby laser on enamel and dentine with a disappointing

7

result. However, the current relationship of dentistry with the laser takes its origins from an article published in 1985 by **Myers and Myers** describing the in vivo removal of dental caries using a modified ophthalmic Nd:YAG laser. Four years later, it was suggested that the Nd:YAG laser could be used for oral soft tissue surgery.

Before the introduction of this wavelength most of the lasers had bulky articulated arms as their delivery systems. It was the first dental laser to use a fiber optic delivery system attached to a small hand piece similar to the size of a dental turbine.

However, with the recent advances and developments of wide range of laser wavelengths and different delivery systems, researchers suggest that lasers could be applied for the dental treatments including periodontal, restorative and surgical treatments.

Since the development of Ruby lasers many types of lasers such as carbon dioxide, Ne:YAG, Argon, Ho:YAG, Er:YAG, Diode lasers etc have evolved in their clinical use .

Unlike many fields of medicine and surgery, where laser treatment represents a sole source of remedy, in dentistry the use of a laser is considered adjunctive in delivering a stage of tissue management conducive to achieving a completed hard or soft tissue procedure.

Essentially, the adjunctive use of surgical lasers in dentistry has sought to address efficient cutting of dental hard tissue, haemostatic ablation of soft tissue and also the sterilising effect through bacterial elimination. Less powerful, non-surgical lasers have been shown to modify cellular activity and enhance biochemical pathways associated with tissue healing, aid in caries detection and assist in the curing of composite restorative materials.

There is growing awareness of the usefulness of laser in the armamentarium of modern dental practice where they can be used as an adjuvant to the traditional approaches[15]. Surprisingly in just one generation

LASER'S have moved out of the realm of fantasy into everyday life from outer space and star wars to compact disc players in our homes to LASER printers & copiers in the office to LASER surgical handpieces with potential to transform the operatory entirely.

HISTORY

Dentistry has entered an exciting era of technology. Today the dental lasers offer dentist not only a window, but a door into this high-tech; rewarding and potentially profitable arena .Pursuit for the advancement in lasers has been going on since ages.

In the early 1900's – Neil Bohr, postulated the "Quantum Mechanics Theory" by overthrowing the till then established 'Light as a Wave front Theory' and suggested that light moved in packets of energy called Quanta. This laid the background for the development of the field of Photonics.

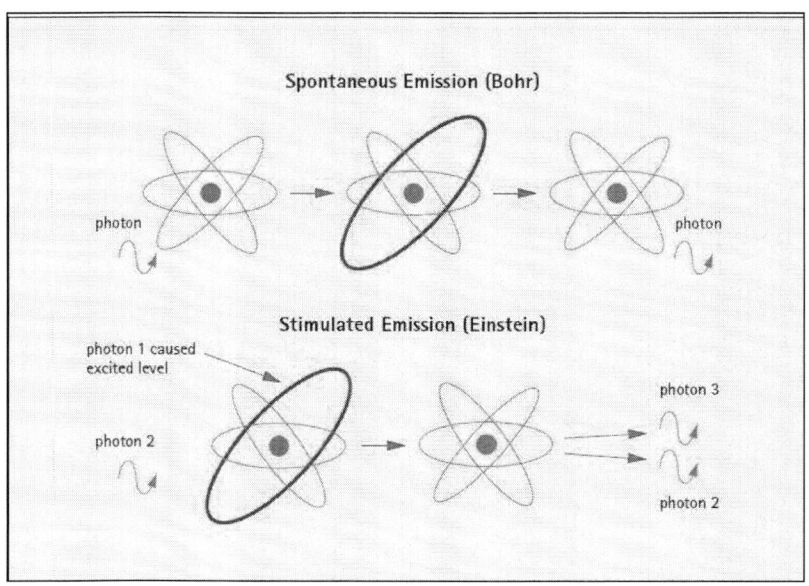

In 1917, an obscure Geneva postal clerk, named **Albert Einstein**, in the International Journal of Physics laid forth a new theory- "Zur Quanta theorie Dur Strahlung" or the "Quantum Theory of Radiation" which was to change the very way we perceive the universe around us and to win its author, Einstein, worldwide fame and the Nobel prize. In this article, he not merely laid the foundation of quantum mechanics, he also postulated on the transmissibility and recovery of energy through the application of photonic emissions. Thus Albert Einstein's celebrated article in 1917 on the stimulated emission of radiation energy is acknowledged as the conceptual basis for amplified light making him the theoretical father of LASER, as Maiman was to develop fame in the future as the practical father of LASER.

In 1955, **C.H.Townes and J.P.Gordon**, two American physicists, in J Physio Rev, reported a new device called the MASER. Townes had simply applied Einstein's quantum mechanics to microwave and had amplified microwave frequencies by the stimulated emission process and had also first coined the term – MASER an acronym for Microwave Amplification by Stimulated Emission of Radiation.

In 1958, Townes CH and a fellow physicist, **Schwanlow Al,** in an article in J Phy Rev, titled 'Infrared And Optical MASERS' discussed the possibility of extending the maser principle to the optical portion and the visible part of the electro-magnetic spectrum. After this article was published, it was an open race against time by many eminent physicists scattered all over the globe, to race in to be the first one to build a device to stimulate light amplification in the visible spectrum.

In 1960, Maiman was the first to have invented LASER, at the Hughes Aircraft Company USA. LASER is an Acronym for (LIGHT AMPLIFICATION BY STIMULATED EMISSION OF RADIATION), using a pulsed ruby laser with a wavelength of (0.694).

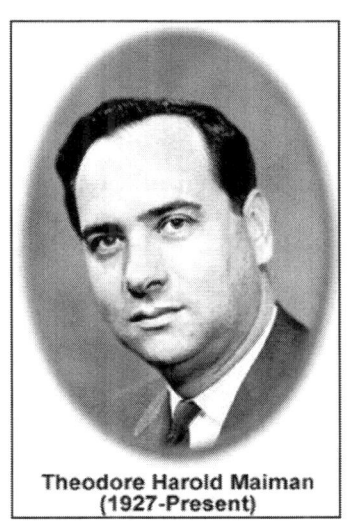

Theodore Harold Maiman
(1927-Present)

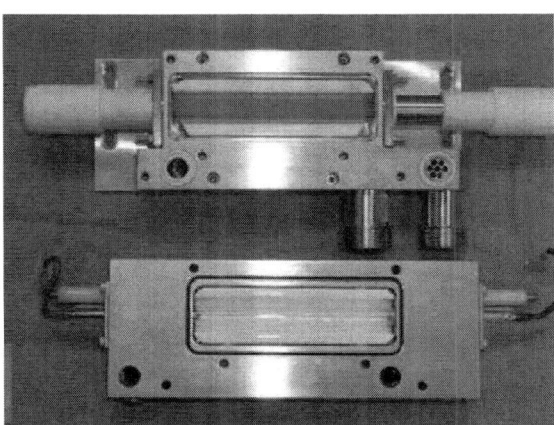

Example of a ruby rod active medium, similar to that used in Maiman's first laser

Within a year of the invention, pioneers such as **Dr Leon Goldman** began research on the interaction of laser light on biologic systems, including early clinical studies on humans. He established the first laser medical laboratory by using a ruby laser to cut, coagulate, ablate and vaporize various biologic tissues. Dr.Goldmann is now honored worldwide, as the first physician to use laser technology, still in its infancy.

11

Interest in medical applications was intense, but the difficulty controlling the power output and delivery of laser energy, together with the relatively poor absorption of these red and infrared wavelengths, led to inconsistent and disappointing results in early experiments.

The exception was the application of the ruby laser in retinal surgery in the mid-1960s.

Many other kinds of laser were invented soon after the solid ruby laser – the first uranium laser by IBM Laboratories (in November 1960), the first helium-neon laser by Bell Laboratories in 1961 and the first semiconductor laser by Robert Hall at General Electric Laboratories in 1962; the first working neodymium- doped yttrium aluminium garnet (Nd:YAG) laser and carbon dioxide laser by Bell Laboratories in 1964, argon ion laser in 1964, chemical laser in 1965 and metal vapour laser in 1966. In each case, the 'name' of the laser was annotated with regard to the active medium (source of laser photons) used.

In 1961 **Snitzer** developed the neodymium laser [22].

Dental research began in 1963 in the University of California at the Los Angles school of Dentistry.

In 1964, the argon ion laser was developed. This continuous wave 488 nm (blue-green) gas laser was easy to control and its high absorption by haemoglobin made it well suited to retinal surgery; clinical systems for treatment of retinal diseases were soon available.

In 1964, **Patel** developed the carbon dioxide lasers [63]. The carbon dioxide laser is a continuous wave gas laser and emits infrared light at 10,600 nm in an easily manipulated, focused beam that is well absorbed by water. Because soft tissue consists mostly of water, researchers found that a carbon dioxide laser beam could cut tissue like a scalpel, but with minimal blood loss. The surgical uses of this laser were investigated extensively from 1967-1970 by pioneers such as **Dr Thomas Polanyi and Geza Jako** and in the early 1970s, use of the carbon dioxide laser in ENT and gynaecologic surgery became well established, but was limited to academic and teaching hospitals.

In the early 1980s, smaller but more powerful lasers became available. Most of these systems were carbon dioxide lasers used for cutting and vaporising tissue and argon lasers for ophthalmic use. These 'second generation' lasers were all continuous wave or CW systems which tend to cause non-selective heat injury, and proper use required a long 'learning curve' and experienced laser surgeons.

The single most significant advance in the use of medical lasers was the concept of 'pulsing' the laser beam, which allowed selective destruction of abnormal or diseased tissue, while leaving surrounding normal tissue undisturbed. The first lasers to fully exploit this principle of selective thermolysis were the pulsed dye lasers introduced in the late 1980s for the treatment of port wine stains in children and shortly after, the first 'Q switched' (ultra-short pulsed) lasers for the treatment of tattoos.

In 1964 **Stern** reported the development of cratering & glasslike fusion of enamel, the penetration and charring of dentin following a single millisecond pulse of ruby laser at 500 to 2000 J/cm^2 & the increased resistance of enamel to acid, which could thus help in caries prevention.

In1965, **Goldman** first reported the exposure of laser done on a vital human tooth and showed that patient experienced no pain with just superficial damage to the crown[33]. In the same year, Taylor et al revealed the effects of Ruby lasers on the dental pulp.

Adrion in 1971 described that the extensive pulpal injury and destruction could occur even with the ruby laser by even at greatly reduced levels[1].

In 1968 **Loben et al** studied the effects of carbon dioxide laser on enamel & dentin which were further explained by **Stern et al** in 1972, by confirming the ability of carbon dioxide to induce resistance to acid penetration of enamel.

In 1974, **Yamamato et al** reported the use of Neodymium: YAG laser in treatment of incipient caries.

In 1977 **Adrion** first used laser welding of Dental Alloys.

Lenz in 1977 reported the use of lasers in Maxillo-facial surgery by creating antral window in maxillary sinus. **Fisher & Frame** of England in 1984 elicited the use of Co_2 laser in excision of benign and pre malignant oral lesions[29]. Wound healing qualities were explained well by **Fisher et al, Pecaro & Gerehime in 1983 & Frame in 1985. Pick et al** in 1985 quoted the effects of carbon dioxide laser & their clinical applications in periodontal surgery[62, 63]. In 1986 Nelson et al discussed the caries precaution through lasers.

Although Maiman had exposed an extracted tooth to his ruby laser in 1960, the possibilities for laser use in dentistry did not occur until 1989, with the production of the American Dental Laser for commercial use. This laser, using an active medium of Nd:YAG, emitted pulsed light and was developed and marketed by Dr. Terry Myers, an American dentist. Though low-powered and due to its emission wavelength, inappropriate for use on dental hard tissue, the availability of a dedicated laser for oral use gained popularity amongst dentists. This laser was first sold in the UK in 1990.

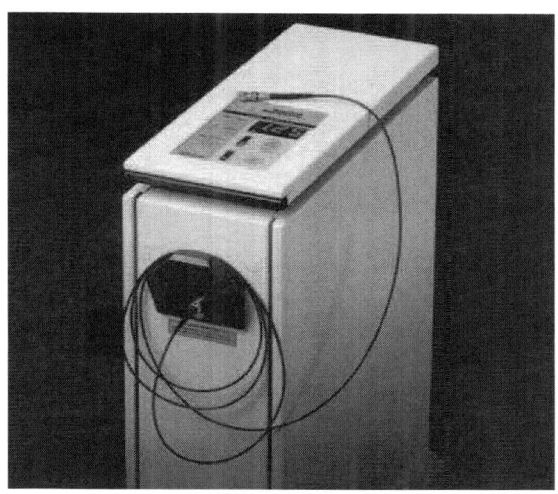

DLase 300 Nd:YAG laser (American Dental Technologies)

Other laser wavelengths, using machines that were already in use in medicine and surgery and only slightly modified, became available for dental use in the early 1990s. Being predominately argon, Nd:YAG, carbon dioxide and semiconductor diodes, all these lasers failed to address a growing need amongst dentists and patients for a laser that would ablate dental hard tissue.

In 1993 **Granados F.J .A et al** studied the advantages of carbon dioxide lasers in treating actinic chelitis and compared with other treatment modalities like cryosurgery, topical application of 5-Fluorouracil, chemical peel with tri-chloroacetic acid, topical application of retinoic acid compounds and vermilionectomy[34].

"**Sexton .J and Hare in 1993**" described the use of argon laser as an ideal tool for the treatment of vascular lesions[73].

In 1997, the FDA, approved the use of pulsed Er:YAG Laser, in the field of dentistry, thus paving the way for widespread commercial manufacture of Er:YAG devices. In the same year, **Cozean .C et al** showed the use of Erbium: YAG laser in human dental cavities such as caries removal, cavity preparation & modification of dentin and enamel before the acid etching for the improved bond strength[22].

In 1998, the FDA Approved the usage of Diode Lasers, a solid state semiconductor laser, with precise energy control and an excellent soft tissue surgical laser for intra-oral use. It has achieved widespread popularity in soft tissue and aesthetic applications.

Kimura .Y et al in 2002 measured the temperature of root surface during root canal preparation using Er:YAG laser irradiation and stated that root canals prepared were clean and almost totally free of debris and smear layer, with open dentinal tubules and no area has melted due laser[47].

Walsh L J in 2003 described the use of low power lasers to elicit a photochemical reaction used to disinfect root canals, periodontal pockets, cavity preparations and sites of peri-implantitis after implant placement[85].

In 2004, **Straus R.A and Fallon S.D** described various types of lasers used in oral and maxillofacial surgery[77]. **Gao et al** in 2006 evaluated the combined effect of carbon dioxide laser and fluoride in inhibiting root demineralization[32]. **Rodrigues et al** in 2006 proved that treatment of enamel by carbon dioxide laser inhibits demineralization in the human mouth and becomes more effective when associated with fluoride[64].

In 2007 **Merchant et al** categorized the lasers and stated that low intensity as well as high intensity lasers can be used for endodontic procedures with low intensity laser used for soft tissues and high intensity lasers for hard tissues[52].

They underlined various endodontic procedures such as disinfection of root canals, sealing of root canals, removal of gutta-percha, laser desensitization, crown lengthening procedures, laser bleaching etc.

Emshoff R et al in 2008 have set up a new land mark in TMJ pain disorder treatment by using low level laser therapy (LLLT) in the management of Temporomandibular Joint pain disorders during function[26].

In February 2009, **Miyakazi. H et al** described the Intra-lesional Photocoagulation (ILP) property of Potassium-titanyl-phosphate (KTP) laser used in the treatment of voluminous vascular lesions in the oral cavity[54].

LASER PHYSICS

Lasers are unique and versatile instruments by virtue of their physical characteristics. There have been different views over the working of lasers and it's important to understand the difference in working and operating methods in order to make an educated decision while choosing a laser for practice.

Surgical lasers are basically the same as scientific or industrial lasers with slight modifications to meet FDA standards and ergonomics of the clinical environment.

Light is a form of energy that exists as a particle called as photon and travels in a wave. 'Ordinary' light refers to the close band of wavelengths in the electromagnetic spectrum that is visible to the human retina. In nature, its origin is in the cosmic stream from space and a common source of man-made ordinary light is the incandescent filament of a light bulb. 'White' light is the sum of all component wavelengths of the visual spectrum. The waveform of ordinary light is non-coherent, in that there is a confused overlap of successive waves. The spread of such waves results in scattering of light with distance and the multi-direction and interference of successive waves gives rise to divergence and dimming with distance. The basic units, or quanta, of light are called **photons.**

There are 3 basic properties of Light[18, 20]:

1. **Velocity** :- Speed of light

2. **Amplitude:** - Measurement of the height of the wave from the zero axis to the peak which describes the energy of that wave.

3. **Wavelength:** - Horizontal distance between any two corresponding points on the wave.

Incident light energy, absorbed by a target atom, will result in an electron moving to a higher energy shell. This unstable state will result in the emission of photonic energy relative to the stable energy state of the target, with excess energy being produced as heat. This is known as spontaneous emission. If an already energized atom is bombarded with a second photon, this will result in the emission of two, coherent photons of identical wavelength. This was postulated by Einstein as stimulated emission.

Laser light occurs through the amplification of stimulated emission. Since the emission energy is unique relative to its source and of known measurable quantity, the light will be of a single wavelength (monochromatic). The precision of the monochromatic beam is due to 'Collimation and Coherence'.

Collimation refers to the beam having specific spatial boundaries. These boundaries ensure that there is a constant beam size and shape that is emitted from the laser unit.

Coherency is a property unique to lasers. The light waves produced by a laser are a specific form of electromagnetic energy. A laser produces light waves that are physically identical, that is, they have identical amplitude and identical frequency.

Hence, a laser produces a monochromatic, collimated and coherent beam of light energy.

In dentistry wavelength ranges between 450-10,600nm. There are 2 gaseous active medium lasers used in dentistry, argon and carbon dioxide. The remainder that are currently available are solid state semiconductor wafers made with multiple layers of metals, such as gallium, aluminum , indium and arsenic or solid rods of garnet crystal grown with various combinations of Yttrium, aluminum, scandium and gallium and then doped with the elements of chromium, neodymium, or erbium.

Quanta of electromagnetic energy are classified as cosmic rays, gamma rays, X-rays, light, microwaves or radio waves. Light may be UV, visible or infra-red. Cosmic rays have extremely short wave length (10-12m) and Radio waves have long wavelength (101m).

Most of the current types of the lasers are classified according to their types of wave length. Short wavelength UV has more energy as compared to the long wavelength infra red lasers.

LIGHT AMPLIFICATION BY STIMULATED EMISSION RADIATION

Thus, the process of lasering occurs when the excited atom can be stimulated to emit photon before the process occurs spontaneously when the photon of exactly right amount of energy enters the electromagnetic field of an excited atom, the incident photon triggers the decay of excited electron to lower energy state which is accompanied by the release of stored energy in the form of second photon.

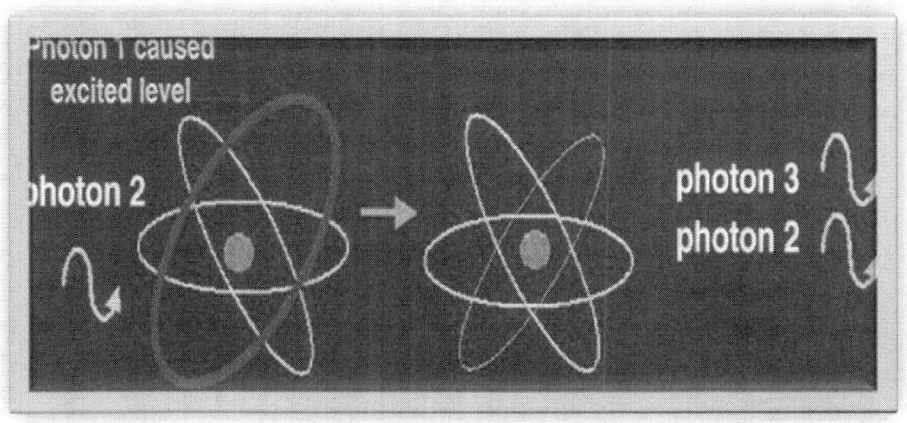

Production of Laser Beam by Photon Excitement

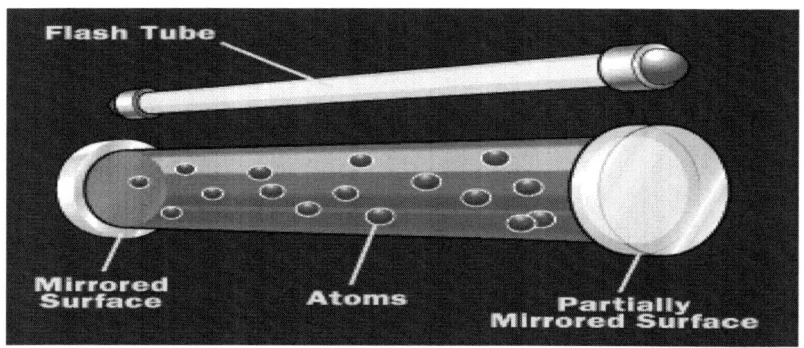

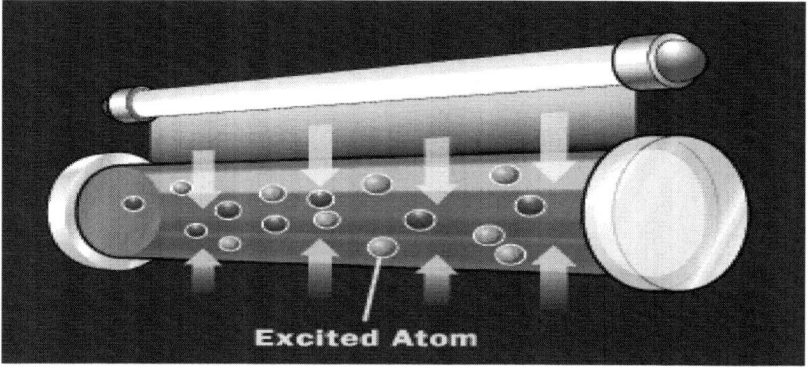

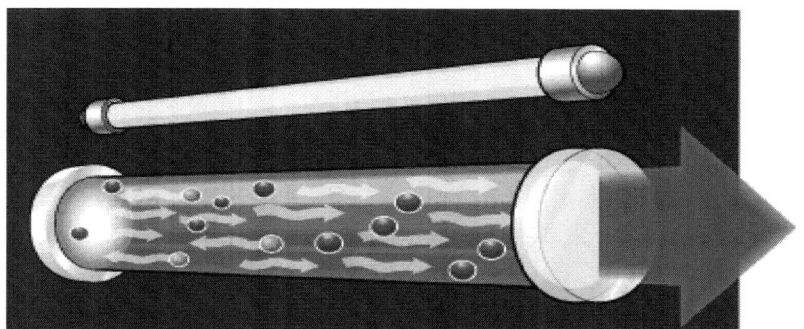

The Process of Amplification

First photon is not absorbed but travels further and excites another atom. Stimulated emission can only occur when the incident photon has exactly the same amount of energy as of the released photon, thus resulting in stimulated emission of two photons of identical wavelength in the same direction.

Release of second photon is time linked to the oscillation of first photon so that photons oscillate together in the phase of a collection of atoms, which includes more number of photons that are pumped into excited state. This is a necessary condition required for lasing. Spontaneous emission of a photon by one atom will stimulate the release of second photon in the second atom & these two photons will trigger the release of two more photons. These four photons yield eight more photons leading to sixteen photons and so on. In the small space, at the speed of light this photon chain reaction produces a brief intense flash of monochromatic light i.e. of the same wavelength & coherent light i.e. of the same phase.

COMPONENTS OF A TYPICAL LASER

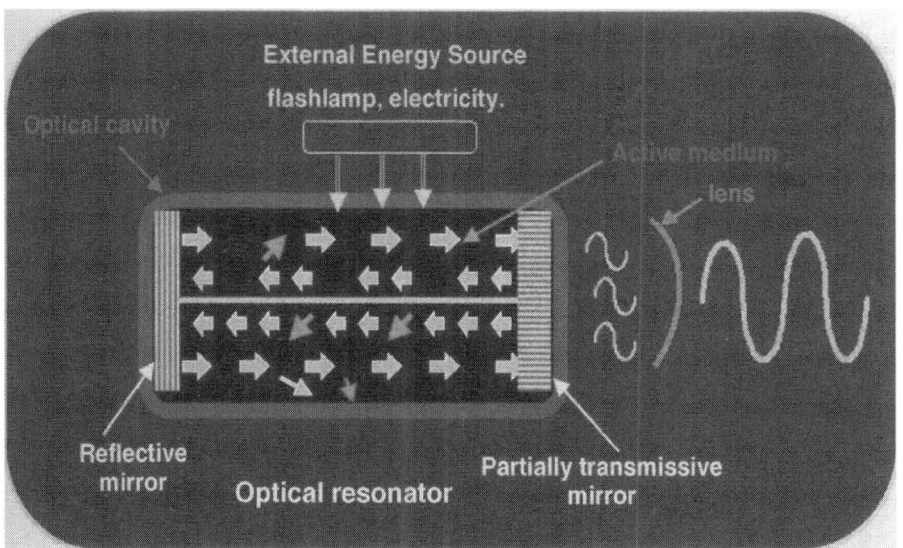

The component parts of a typical laser are:

1. **ACTIVE MEDIUM** -A material, either naturally occurring or man-made that when stimulated, emits laser light. This lasing medium determines the wavelength of the light emitted from the laser. It is the most important component because this type of medium denotes the name of the laser systems. For e.g. If carbon dioxide is used as a lasing medium, it is known as carbon dioxide laser.

This material may be a solid, liquid or gas. The first 'dental' laser used a crystal of neodymium-doped yttrium aluminium garnet (Nd:YAG) as its active medium. 'YAG' is a complex crystal with the chemical composition $Y_3Al_5O_{12}$. During crystal growth, 1% neodymium ($Nd3+$) ions are doped into the YAG crystal. Other lasers of significance in dentistry use rare earth and other metal ions within a 'doped' YAG crystal lattice, eg erbium (Er: YAG) and holmium (Ho:YAG), together with another erbium and chromium-doped garnet of yttrium, scandium and gallium (Er,Cr: YSGG). The active medium is positioned within the laser cavity, an internally-polished tube, with mirrors co-axially positioned at each end and surrounded by the external energising input, or pumping mechanism. The 'active medium', e.g. carbon dioxide, Nd:YAG, defines the type of laser and the emission wavelength of the laser (10,600 nm and 1,064 nm respectively). Atoms of the active medium are absorbed by the process of light emission.

2. **PUMPING MECHANISM** - This represents a man-made source of primary energy that excites the active medium. It excites or pumps the atom in the laser medium to their higher energy levels. This causes the "Population Inversion". It happens when there are more atoms in the excited state pumped by the electrical charge rather than a non-excited state. Atoms in the excited state spontaneously emit photons of light, which bounce back and forth between the two mirrors in the laser tube. As they bounce within the laser tube, they strike other atoms, stimulating more spontaneous emission. Photons of energy of the same wavelength and frequency escape through the transmissive mirror as the laser beam.

This is usually a light source, either a flashlight or arc-light, but can be a diode laser unit or an electromagnetic coil. Energy from this primary source is absorbed by the active medium, resulting in the production of laser light. This process is very inefficient, with only some 3-10% of incident energy resulting in laser light, the rest being converted to heat energy. The dynamics of incident energy with time has a fundamental bearing on the emission mode characteristics of a given laser. A continuous- feed electrical discharge will result in a similar continuous feed of laser light emission.

3. **OPTICAL RESONATOR** - Laser light produced by the stimulated active medium is bounced back and forth through the axis of the laser cavity, using two mirrors placed at either end, thus amplifying the power. The distal mirror is totally reflective and the proximal mirror is partly transmissive, so that at a given energy density, laser light will escape to be transmitted to the target tissue.

4. **DELIVERY SYSTEM** - The coherent collimated bean of laser light must be able to be delivered to the target tissue in manner that is ergonomic and precise. Light can be delivered by a numbered of different mechanisms. Several years ago, a hand held laser meant holding a larger; several hundred pounds laser usually the size of desk above a patient. Although the idea was comical at the time, technological advances are producing smaller and lighter weight lasers.

Dependent upon the emitted wavelength, the delivery system may be a quartz fibre-optic, a flexible hollow waveguide, an articulated arm (incorporating mirrors), or a hand-piece containing the laser unit (at present only for low powered lasers).

Articulated arms : Laser light can be delivered by articulated arms, which are very simple but elegant devices. Mirrors are placed at 45° angles to tubes carrying the laser light. The tubes can rotate about the normal axis of the mirrors. This results in a tremendous amount of flexibility in the arm and in delivering the laser light. This is typically used with carbon dioxide laser. The arm does have some disadvantages that include the arms counter weight and the limited ability to move in straight line.

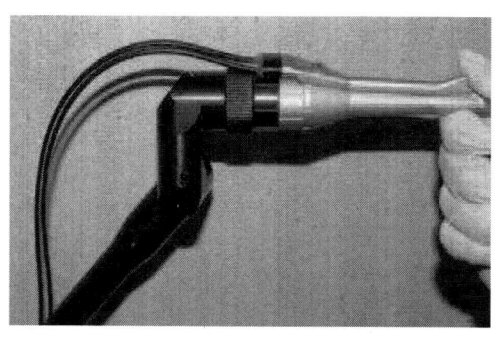

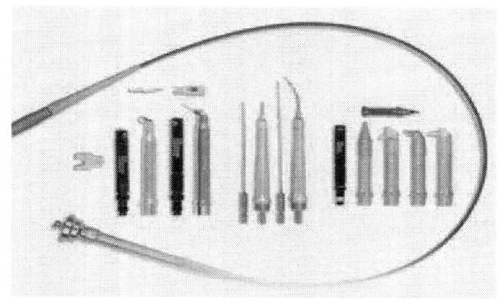

Articulated Arm and Hollow Waveguide

Before the introduction of Nd:YAG lasers in 1990 most of the dental lasers used bulky articulated arms as their delivery systems. These articulated arms were not conducive to the practice of general dentistry due to long learning curve needed to master their use and the difficulty in the delivery of laser energy to the entire oral cavity[44]. But, the latest articulated arms used are user friendly and easier to manage.

Optical fiber: Laser light can be delivered by an optical fiber, which is frequently used with near infrared and visible lasers. The light is trapped in the glass and propagates down through the fiber in a process called "Total Internal Reflection". This cable can be more pliant than the waveguide, has a corresponding decrease in weight and resistance to movement, and is usually smaller in diameter (some soft tissue lasers have optic fibers with sizes ranging from 200-600μm). Although the glass component is encased in a resilient sheath, it can be fragile and cannot be bent into a sharp angle. The fiber fits snugly into a handpiece with the bare end protruding or, in the case of the erbium family of lasers, with an attached sapphire or quartz tip. There are certain disadvantages of optical fibers such as:-

1. The beam is no longer collimated when emitted from the fiber. The light diverges at some angle, which limits the focal spot size.
2. The light is no longer coherent.

The Nd:YAG laser was the first dental laser to use a fiber-optic delivery system attached to a small handpiece similar in size to the dental turbine. This made the delivery of laser energy to every part of the oral cavity a much easier process.

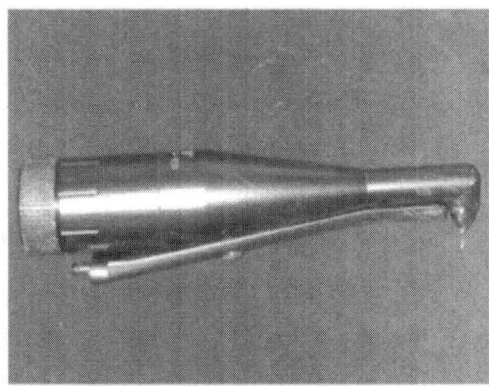

Er: YAG Handpiece with Optical Fiber

In the non surgical periodontal procedures, the optical fibers used to deliver the laser energy are only end-lasing fibers; that is, the energy comes out only from fiber tip but not along the side walls of the fiber.

This fiber system can be used contact or non-contact mode. Most of the time it is used in contact fashion directly touching the surgical site.

All the conventional dental instruments, hand or rotary physically touch the tissues being treated, giving the operator instant feedback. Dental lasers can be used in contact or out of contact. Clinically, a laser used out of contact can provide easy access to otherwise difficult to reach areas of tissue. For example a fiber tip can be used around the lining of a periodontal pocket to remove small amounts of granulation tissue. When used out of contact, the beam is aimed a few millimeters away from the target. This modality is useful for various tissue contours, but the loss of tactile sensation demands that surgeon pays close attention to the tissue interaction with the laser energy. All the invisible dental lasers are equipped with a separate aiming beam, which can be laser or conventional light. The aiming beam is delivered coaxially along the fiber or waveguide and shows the operator the spot, where the laser energy will be focused.

In either modality, lenses within the laser instrument focus the beam. With the hollow waveguide, there is a spot of a specific diameter where the beam is in sharp focus and where the energy is the greatest. That spot, called the focal point, should be used for incisional and excisional surgery. For the optic fiber and accessories, the focal point is at or near the tip, which has the greatest energy. In either case, the beam becomes divergent and defocused as the handpiece is moved away from the focal point. At a small divergent distance, the laser light can cover a wider area, which is useful is achieving hemostasis. At a greater distance, the beam loses its effectiveness because the energy dissipates, with a proportional decrease in power density.

Thus, suitability of the delivery system is conditional upon the emission wavelength of the laser. Therefore, lasers with shorter wavelengths, such as argon, diodes and Nd:YAG can be designed with small flexible glass fibers. Whereas Er, Cr:YSGG, Er:YAG and carbon dioxide lasers, present challenges to fibre because there wavelengths are large and do not fit easily into the crystalline molecules of the conducting glass. Additionally they are highly absorbed into water, so a special and costly fibre design with a structure of minimal hydroxyl content, incorporating peripheral cooling air and water spray for the hand piece is necessary. Hence they require alternative delivery systems, such as articulated arms incorporating internal mirrors and prisms, and hollow waveguides, where the light is reflected along internally-polished tubes. Newer, water-free fibre compounds, e.g. zirconium fluoride, are being developed to overcome this problem.

5. **COOLING SYSTEM** - Heat production is a by-product of laser light propagation. It increases with the power output of the laser and hence, with heavy-duty tissue cutting lasers, the cooling system represents the bulkiest component. Co-axial coolant systems may be air- or water assisted.

6. **CONTROL PANEL** - This allows variation in power output with time, above that defined by the pumping mechanism frequency. Other facilities may allow wavelength change (multi-laser instruments) and print-out of delivered laser energy during clinical use.

MODE OF DELIVERY OF THE LASER

Often, a clinical laser is referred to as 'continuous wave' (CW), 'gated pulsed' (GP) or 'free-running pulsed' (FRP). Although this might appear confusing, it relates to the rate of emission of laser light with time. The inherent benefit of the concept of pulsed flow over average continuous flow is that, assuming the average delivery of energy with time might be low, the peak-energy of each 'pulse' can be significantly higher.

The important principle of any laser device is that light energy strikes the tissue for a certain length of time, producing a thermal interaction. If the laser uses a pulsed emission mode, either gated or free running, the targeted tissue has some time to cool before the next pulse of light energy is emitted. In continuous wave mode, the surgeon must manually cease laser emission periodically to allow thermal relaxation to occur. If an excessive thermal energy is applied, healing is delayed and increased post-operative discomfort occurs.

Thin or fragile soft tissues like those to be lased in periodontal therapies or in muco-gingival surgeries, i.e. Aberrant Frenulum, should always be treated by a pulsed mode, so that the amount and rate of tissue removal is smaller and slower and there is minimal chance of irreversible thermal damage to the target and the adjacent non target tissues. Longer intervals between pulses can also help to avoid the transfer of deleterious heat to the surrounding tissues.

For thick fibrous tissues, as for example in Gingivectomies done in Idiopathic Gingival Enlargements, the tissue is dense and requires more energy for rapid, yet safe speed of excision. Also a gentle air stream or water current helps in keeping the target area cooler. Hence, a continuous wave emission device is an ideal choice for these clinical conditions.

In practice, the emission mode for any given laser can be either **'inherent' or 'acquired'**. Inherent emission modes are related to the nature of the excitation source:

a) Free-running pulsed, where laser emission occurs over a pulse width of 100-200 microseconds.

b) Continuous wave.

Acquired emission modes are due to a modifying effect (electrical, mechanical, electro-optical or acousto-optical) acting upon the inherent delivery:

a) Chopped or gated CW, where laser emission occurs over tenths (0.1-0.5) of a second.

b) Q-switched, mode-locked (not applicable in dental lasers).

c) Super-pulsed, where laser emission occurs over 300-400 microseconds.

Once the laser is produced, its output power may be delivered in the following modes :

CONTINUOUS MODE

This was the first developed emission mode and this delivery technology is still to be found in older laser devices. On activation by pressing the foot switch, the laser beam is emitted at one power level continuously as a wave as long as the foot switch is kept depressed. When laser machines are set in a continuous wave mode, the amplitude of the output beam is expressed in terms of watts. The laser emits radiation continuously at a constant power level of between 10 to 100W. The carbon dioxide laser is the most commonly used laser in general surgery. It can be operated as a continuous wave laser by maintaining a continuous discharge through the gas which acts as a medium.

CHOPPED MODE

A shutter that "chops" the beam into trains of short pulses can interrupt the output of a continuous wave laser. This is mainly done either electrically or mechanically. Such units are based upon a continuous wave diode or He:Ne base unit which can be chopped to give a pseudo pulsing effect. With the output chopped in such a way the unit's average radiant power is dropped dramatically. The maximum power level of each pulse is same as that obtained in the continuous wave mode. The speed of the shutter is 100 to 500ms (microseconds) or thousandth of a second [1×10^{-6}]. Where such units allow for alteration of the pulse repetition rate, two important characteristics of emitted output will change with changes in the pulse repetition rate:

a) The pulse width or duration varies, usually decreasing with increasing pulse repetition rate.

b) The average radiant power output falls as the pulse repetition rate is increased.

GATED OR PULSED MODE

Lasers can be gated or pulsed electronically. This type of gating permits the duration of the pulses to be compressed, producing a corresponding increase in peak power that is much higher than in commonly available in the continuous wave mode. Surgical lasers have a mechanical shutter positioned in the beam path (like a camera).

A timing circuit controls the opening and closing of the shutter. Timing values are set by controls on the front panel console. The time sequence is activated when the user steps on the foot pedal, or in some units, presses the button on the handpiece. Single pulses can have duration such as 0.05, 0.1, 0.2, 0.5, and 1.0 sec, or the shutter can remain open as long as the pedal is depressed (continuous). Timing circuits vary in sophistication. Usually pulse duration can be set and the time between pulses can be varied independently, changing the repetition rate. On some units, bursts of pulses can be delivered.

SUPER PULSED MODE & ULTRA PULSED MODE

The term super pulsed mode is used to describe the output of a gated high peak power laser with short pulse duration typically between hundreds of microseconds ($1ms = 1 \times 10^{-6}$ seconds). The pulse produced during super pulsing can have a repetition rate of 50 to 250 pulses per second that permits the laser output to appear almost continuous during use.

Ultra pulsed mode produces an output pulse of high peak power that is maintained for a longer time and delivers more energy in each pulse and the duration of the ultra pulse is slightly less as compared to the super pulsed mode.

FLASH LAMP PULSING

In these systems, a flash lamp is used to pump the lasing medium, usually for solid state lasers (e.g. Nd:YAG). As with the pulsed carbon dioxide peak powers are higher since the energy is confined to short duration pulses. The duration of the flash lamp, typically 0.1 to 0.8 m sec (100 to 800- μsec), determines the duration of the output pulse.

Q-SWITCHING

Shorter duration pulses are achieved with Q-switching lasers. A simple Q-switch uses two components not used in any of the other laser systems, an optimal polarizer and a pocket cell.

There is a rotating mirror which is used as a part of the optical cavity. Only when the rotating mirror is precisely aligned with the output mirror, is lasing possible. Lasing is restricted to a very short time interval (1-10 nanoseconds). The Q-switch components allow a tremendous amount of energy to build up with in the optical cavity before it is released in a short powerful burst. Thus, several hundred mill joules of energy can be squeezed into nanosecond pulsed.

The three different types of Q-switched lasers are used in dentistry, these are :-

- ➢ Ruby lasers
- ➢ Neodymium:Yttrium-Aluminium-Gartnet Laser
- ➢ Alexandrite laser

FOCUSED / DEFOCUSED MODE

Lasers can be used in either a focused mode or defocused mode. A focused mode is made when the laser beam hits the tissue at its focal point (or) smallest diameter. (This diameter is dependent on the size of lens used). This mode can also be referred to as the cutting mode.

In the defocused mode, laser beam is moved away from the focal plane. The beam size that hits the tissue has a greater diameter, thus causing a wider area of tissue to be vaporized. However, the laser intensity of the power density is reduced. This mode is also known as the ablation mode.

CONTACT AND NON-CONTACT MODES

In contact mode, the fiber handpiece is placed in contact to the tissue whereas in the non-contact mode, the handpiece is placed away from the target tissue. In non-contact mode, the clinician operates with visual control with the aid of an aiming beam or by observing the tissue effect being created. Several modes are available for achieving pulsed output from a continuous wave laser.

These are:-

a) Mode Locking

Method of clipping avalanche of wavelength reflected back and forth between the mirrors in synchronism with reciprocating travel of these wavelengths in the optical cavity so that only those wavelengths which have intensity above a certain threshold are transmitted. Synchronization of wavelength is achieved by the use of a shutter or bleachable dye. Mode of locking produces pulses with a high peak power from a Pico-second to Nano-second duration.

b) Q-Switching :-

Shorter duration pulses are derived from the Q-switching. It uses a rotary mirror as a part of optical cavity. Only when the optical mirror is precisely aligned with the output mirror lasing is possible, so lasing is restricted to a very short interval (1-10 nsec)

c) Cavity Dumping:-

Creates large population inversion and a condition of strong resonance in the optical cavity, but does not allow any of the coherent light to escape from resonator except when an electroscopic switch is activated. The light then emerges from laser in a pulse of short duration and high intensity.

d) Pump Pulsing :-

This is a method of cyclically or intermittently interrupting the flow of power from the pumping source into the laser resonator of mechanical , electric, electronically or electro-optical switching device according to the form of energy used for pumping the laser medium. Produces output that ranges from 10-100 times as high as maximum continuous wave power obtainable from the same laser. This kind of pulsing is most commonly used in surgical lasers.

PROPERTIES OF LASERS [30, 36]

These are:-

- ➤ **Monochromatic :** Light is emitted at one or more single wavelengths with a very narrow line width & they are of the same frequency wavelength & energy[18].
- ➤ **Coherent :** Wavelength is perfectly in step with the rest of the beam, both laterally & longitudinally i.e. the waves produced are of identical wavelength and frequency.
- ➤ **Collimation :** - It is a ray of single divergence i.e the beam has specific spatial boundaries with constant beam size and shape emitted from laser unit[14].

According to the different properties of lasers as well as the properties of material, effect of lasers on tissues or its interaction with photons are enlisted as :-

- ➤ Thermal interactions
- ➤ Photo chemical interactions
- ➤ Non – linear processes

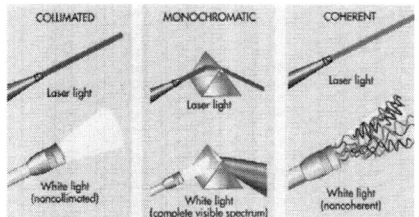

Properties of Lasers

TISSUE INTERACTION OF LASERS[30]

LASER TISSUE INTERACTION	
TISSUE INTERACTIONS	TYPES OF LASERS
PHOTOTHERMAL	Carbon dioxide, Nd:YAG, Er:YAG
PHOTODISRUPTION	Nd:YAG, Dye(pulsed)
PHOTOABLATION	Excimer,Er:YAG,Carbon dioxide(pulsed)
PHOTODYNAMIC	Dye, Metal Vapor
BIOSTIMULATION	He:Ne, Diodes

The light energy from a laser can have four different interactions with the target tissue, and these interactions depend on the optical properties of that tissue and the wavelength used.

These are [9, 18, 21, 86]:-

- ➤ Absorption
- ➤ Reflection
- ➤ Transmission
- ➤ Scattering

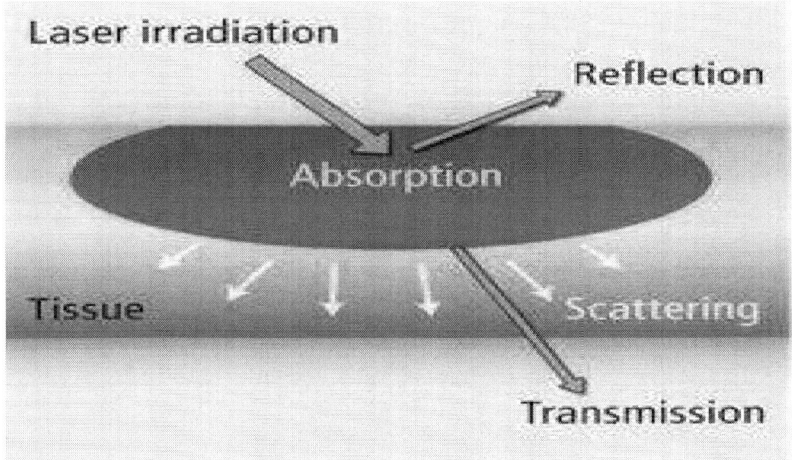

ABSORPTION:-

This interaction is of laser energy by the intended target tissue. This effect is the usual desirable effect, and the amount of energy that is absorbed by the tissue depends on the tissue characteristics, such as pigmentation and water content, and on the laser wavelength and emission mode. Certain wavelengths are absorbed preferentially by certain tissue compounds called the chromophores. In general, the shorter wavelengths, from about 500 to 1000 nm, are absorbed readily in pigmented tissue. Hemoglobin, the molecule that transports oxygen to tissues reflects red wavelengths, imparting color to arterial blood. It therefore is strongly absorbed by blue and green wavelengths. Venous blood, containing less oxygen, absorbs more red light and appears darker. The pigment melanin, which imparts color to skin is strongly absorbed by short wavelengths. Water, the universally present molecule, has varying degrees of absorption by different wavelengths.

Dental structures have different amounts of water content by weight. A ranking from lowest to highest would show enamel (with 2%-3%), dentin, bone, calculus, caries, and soft tissue (at about 70%). Hydroxyapatite is the chief crystalline component of dental hard tissues and has a wide range of absorption depending on the wavelength. In general, the shorter wavelengths from about 500 to 1000nm are absorbed more readily in pigmented tissues and blood elements. Argon has a high affinity for melanin and hemoglobin in soft tissue. Diode and Nd:YAG have a high affinity for melanin and less interaction with hemoglobin. The longer wavelengths are more interactive with water and

hydroxyapatite. Erbium is well absorbed by hydroxyapatite and water. Carbon dioxide is well absorbed by water and has the greatest affinity for tooth structure.

REFLECTION:-

 In this type of interaction beam redirects itself off of the tissue surface, having no effect on the target tissue. A caries detecting laser device uses the reflected light to measure the degree of sound tooth structure. The reflected light could maintain its collimation property in a narrow beam or become more diffuse. The laser beam generally becomes more divergent as the distance from the handpiece increases. The beam from some lasers can still have adequate energy at distances greater than 3 m, however. This reflection can be dangerous because the energy would be directed to an unintentional target, such as the eyes[9]. This causes a major safety concern for dental laser use in the operatory.

TRANSMISSION:-

This interaction is of the laser energy directly through the tissue, with no effect on the target tissue. It is highly dependent on the wavelength of laser light. Water, for example, is relatively transparent to the shorter wavelengths such as diode, argon and Nd:YAG, whereas tissue fluids readily absorb the erbium family and carbon dioxide at the outer surface so that there is little energy transmitted to adjacent tissues. An Nd:YAG laser would work better in an environment difficult to keep dry, whereas a carbon dioxide laser would be less effective because of its absorption by saliva, water, and tissue fluids. As another example, the diode and Nd:YAG lasers can be transmitted through the lens, iris, cornea, anterior chamber, posterior chamber, vitreous, and aqueous humors of the eye without affecting them, yet can be absorbed easily by the tissues of the retina.

SCATTERING:-

Scattering is shown by the change in direction of the radiation without loss of energy. This change in direction is the result of the encounter of the ray with small particles or molecules. The directional character is lost and the irradiated volume becomes larger, dissipating the thermal effects. This fourth interaction of the laser light, that is scattering, causes weakening of the intended energy and possibly producing no useful biologic effect. Scattering of the laser beam causes the heat transfer to the tissues adjacent to the surgical site, and thus the unwanted thermal damage can occur. However, a beam deflected in different directions would be useful in facilitating the curing of composite resins and in covering a broad area.

The primary and beneficial effect of laser energy is absorption of the laser light by the intended biologic tissue. Dental laser surgery optimizes these photobiologic effects. Incisions and excisions with accompanying precision and hemostasis are one of the many advantages of lasers.

Besides photothermal effects, there are other effects of lasers on selected tissues. These are photochemical effects that lasers create to stimulate chemical reactions, such as the curing of composite resins. Lasers also can act photochemically to break chemical bonds, such as in the process of photodynamic therapy, a new addition to the armamentarium of oncologists for treating cancer. Lasers may also have photoacoustic effects in which the pulse of laser energy on hard dental tissues can produce a shock wave, which then explodes or pulverizes the tissue, creating an abraded crater[85].

THERMAL EFFECTS OF LASERS [16]

TISSUE TEMP	OBSERVED EFFECT
37-50°C	HYPERTHERMIA.
> 60° C	COAGULATION, PROTEIN DENATURATION.
70-90°C	WELDING OF TISSUES.
100-150°C	VAPORIZATION .
> 200°C	CARBONIZATION.

The thermal effects of laser energy primarily revolve around the water content of the tissues and the temperature rise of the tissues. When the tissue temperature reaches approximately 60^0C, proteins begin to denature without any vaporization of the underlying tissue. Hence this temperature range is useful for removing granulation tissue. Coagulation refers to the irreversible damage to the tissue and this process produces the desirable effect of hemostasis. Soft tissue edges can be welded together with a uniform heating to 70^0C, to 80^0C. When the target tissue is elevated to a temperature of 100^0C, vaporization of water within the tissues occurs, a process called as ablation. Because soft tissues are composed of a high percentage of water, excision of soft tissue begins at this temperature. Hence, a temperature range of 100^0 -150^0 C is ideal for Gingivoplasties, Gingivectomies and Frenotomies. When the tissue temperature is raised to about 200^0C, it is dehydrated and then burned in the presence of air. Carbon as an end product, absorbs all wavelengths. This causes a great deal of collateral thermal damage over a wider area.

LASER TYPES

A varied number and variety of lasers are being put to use in dentistry today. On a broad basis they can be classified as follows:

According to **Frentzen.M & Koort.H.J (1990)**[30]

BASED ON THE TYPE OF DELIVERY SYSTEM:

- ➤ Flexible hollow wave guide / articulating arms.
- ➤ Glass fiber optic cable

BASED ON THE TYPE OF LASER MEDIUM USED:

- ➤ Gas
- ➤ Solid
- ➤ Liquid

BASED ON TYPE OF INTERACTION WITH TISSUE:

According to Baurele.D (1994) & Berlien.H.P et al (1989)[10]

- ➤ Contact lasers
- ➤ Non-contact lasers

BASED ON THE TYPE OF APPLICATION [74, 76] :

According to Smith.P.W et al & Strang. R et al (1988)

➢ Soft tissue lasers: Low power lasers, about 1000mW

➢ Hard tissue lasers: high power, about 3 W or more

SOFT TISSUE LASERS:

Soft lasers are a low power lasers which emit in the visible or near infrared region of the spectrum These are a new therapeutic tool to be used in dentistry. The use of soft tissue lasers to augment conventional dental therapy has increased dramatically in recent years[74].

Biological effects :

- Increased pain tolerance due to changes in cell membrane potential

- Vasodilatation leading to improved metabolism

- Earlier resolution of edema

- Immuno-stimulation

- Accelerated intracellular metabolism, e.g. activation of enzymes

- Overall stimulation of soft tissue healing by selectively influencing connective tissue metabolism

Uses :

Soft laser therapy has been recommended for the following dental conditions:

- Oral ulceration, Periodontal diseases

- Alveolitis, Herpes labialis

- Pericoronitis, Pulpitis

- De-pigmentation, Vascular lesions
- Nausea induced by dental procedures[27, 34, 73, 74].

HARD TISSUE LASERS:

These are the solid state pulsed lasers that have maximum emission at mid-infrared spectrum. These wavelengths correspond to the peak absorption range of water in the infrared spectrum[85].

Biological effects [11] :

- Crazing, Cratering[33, 87]
- Glazing, Enamel & dentin ablation
- Inhibition of demineralization

Uses:

- Laser fluorescence detection of caries
- Laser fluorescence detection of sub-gingival calculus
- Caries removal
- Cavity preparation, Re-mineralization
- Arthroscopic surgical procedures
- Curing light activated materials, Laser etching[85,87]

LASER WAVELENGTHS USED IN DENTISTRY

According to **Frentzen.M & Koort.H.J** in 1990 types of laser according to the different wavelength and different emission modes are:-

TYPES OF LASERS ACCORDING TO THE DIFFERENT WAVELENGTHS			
LASER	WAVELENGTH	MODE	POWER
CO_2	9000-11000	CW,PULSED	UP TO 1000
Er:YAG	2940	PULSED	UP TO 10
HO:YAG	2100	PULSED	UP TO 10
Nd:YAG	1064+1300	CW,PULSED	UP TO 500
DIODES	650-950	PULSED	UP TO 10
He:Ne	633	CW	UP TO .08
DYES	450-1200	CW,PULSED	UP TO 10
Ar ION	488+514	CW	UP TO 30
EXCIMER	190-351	PULSED	UP TO 100

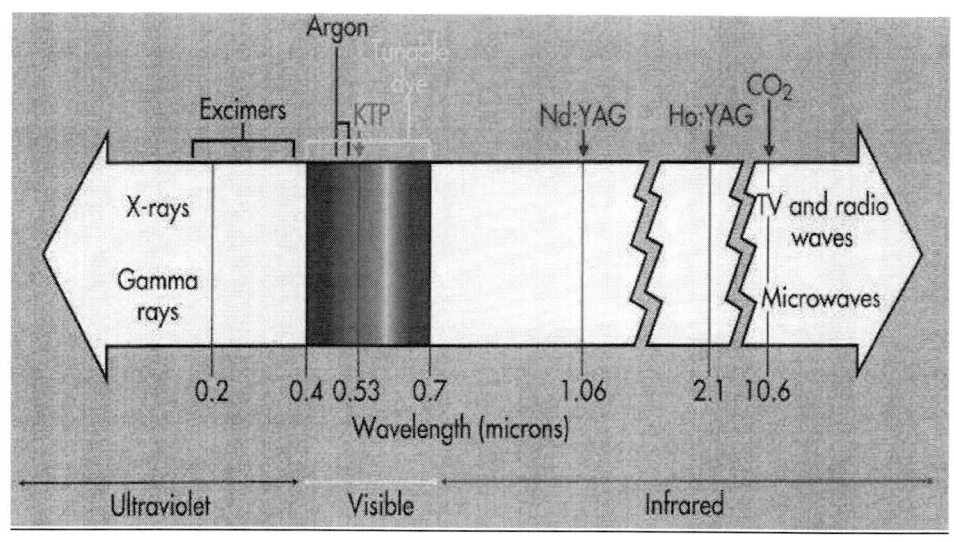

TYPES OF LASERS AND THEIR USES:-

Frentzen .M & Koort.H.J in 1990 described the types of lasers according to their delivery systems[30]

DELIVERY SYSTEMS FOR LASERS	
LASER	DELIVERY SYSTEM
Carbon Dioxide	Mirror system,fibers in development
Er:YAG	Mirror system,fibers in development
Ho:YAG	Fiber system
Diodes	Fiber system
He:Ne	Fiber system
Dyes	Fiber system
Ar ion	Fiber system
Excimer	Mirror system, fibers in development

CARBON DIOXIDE LASER[20, 21, 63, 86]

- ➢ 1964, **Patel et al**

- ➢ Carbon dioxide lasers emit radiation in the mid-infrared portion of the spectrum at a wavelength of 10,600 nm.

- ➢ This laser uses a mixture of carbon dioxide, nitrogen, and helium as its medium.

- ➢ This medium is usually excited by a high voltage electrical current. Because the photons from this laser cannot be transmitted in a fiber-optic cable, it is necessary to deliver the beam to one of the available hand pieces.

- ➢ CO_2 lasers are invisible, so a red helium neon laser is used in parallel or near parallel, as an aiming beam.

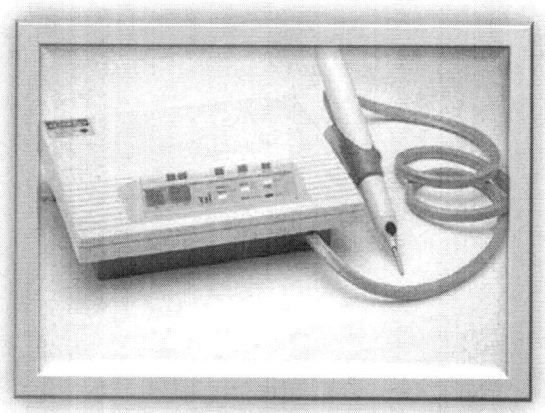

The different types of delivery modes can be used for CO_2 lasers such as:-

a) Continuous mode: Emits constant beam of energy as operator steps on the pedal.

b) Regular pulsing mode: operator can set the number of pulses.

c) Super-pulsing: Short, high-powered pulses

d) Ultra pulsing or Flash scanning : Short, high-powered pulses

➢ Carbon dioxide lasers reflect off mirrors, allowing access to difficult areas. Unfortunately, they also reflect off dental instruments, making accidental reflection to non-target tissue a concern.

➢ Carbon dioxide lasers cannot be delivered fiber optically. Advances in articulated arms and hollow wave-guide technologies now provide easy access to all areas of the mouth.

➢ Regardless of the delivery method used, all carbon dioxide lasers work in a non-contact mode. Of all the lasers for oral use, carbon dioxide is the fastest in removing tissue.

➢ The chromophore that absorbs the carbon dioxide wavelength is water, the carbon dioxide laser is the most commonly used laser in the oral cavity.

➢ Depth of penetration can be as shallow as 0.2mm, with little scatter, reflection or transmission.

Uses:

❖ This laser is readily absorbed by water and therefore is very effective for the surgery of soft tissues, which have a high water content. The primary advantage of carbon dioxide laser surgery over the scalpel is the strong hemostatic and bactericidal effect.

❖ Very little wound contraction and minimal scarring are other advantages of laser surgery, especially for the carbon dioxide laser.

❖ Carbon dioxide lasers are effective and most commonly used by oral and maxillofacial surgeons in removal of benign tumors and pre-malignant lesions.

❖ These are commonly used for excision and ablation of various types of superficial lesions and for skin resurfacing.

❖ This laser destroys the viability of calculus & microbial plaque deposits **Cobb et al, 1977** but does not remove calculus from root surface.

❖ Adjunct to mechanical root instrumentation **Tucker, Cobb & Rapley 1996**.

❖ Its use is limited to soft tissue procedures; in hard tissues – cracking, melting & carbonization. **Lobene et al, 1968.**

❖ In pulsed & defocused mode at low energy output this laser may have root conditioning, detoxification & bactericidal effect on the contaminated root surfaces.

Basic and Clinical Studies:

➢ **Tucker et al.**[82] evaluated the effects of the carbon dioxide laser on calculus in vitro and reported that the pulsed carbon dioxide laser at 6 W and 20 Hz (pulse duration: 0.01 s) was able to remove dental plaque on the root surface, whereas only melting and carbonization occurred on the dental calculus of extracted teeth.

➤ **Baron et al.**[8] investigated the effects of the pulsed defocus mode carbon dioxide laser. The carbon dioxide laser at 2.0 W and 4 Hz with 4.0 mm spot size did not result in any extensive damages to the root surface, which was flat and smooth with apparent fusion of the smear layer. They concluded that the pulsed defocus mode may present the advantage of decontaminating the root surface.

➤ **Crepsi et al.**[23] reported that after the pulsed defocus mode carbon dioxide laser treatment at 2 W and 1 Hz, the periodontally diseased root surface showed the highest number of tightly attached fibroblasts compared with the nontreated control and scaling and root planing (SRP) alone. They concluded that pulsed defocus mode carbon dioxide laser treatment combined with mechanical instrumentation constitutes a useful tool for root conditioning.

➤ **Coffelt et al**[12] found that, when used at an energy density between 11 and 41 mJ/cm2 in the defocused mode, the carbon dioxide laser destroyed microbial colonies without inflicting undue damage to the root surfaces. Thus, the carbon dioxide laser, when used with high-energy output, especially in a continuous wave mode, is not appropriate for calculus removal and root surface debridement due to major thermal side-effects, such as carbonization. However, when used with relatively low energy output in a pulsed and/or defocused mode, this laser may have root conditioning, detoxification and bactericidal effects on the contaminated root surfaces.

ARGON LASER[21, 73, 86]

➤ It was first developed at aircraft research laboratories by **"Bridges in 1964".**

➤ The conventional argon laser delivers a green- blue light beam in the 488 or 514nm range and is activated by the electrical current. It is the only soft tissue laser that operates within the visible portion of the electromagnetic spectrum.

➤ This can be used with a fiber-optic cable and hand piece & it can be used in the continuous mode using a contact delivery system.

> In oral tissues there is no reflection, but some absorption, some scattering and transmission is seen.

> The visible blue-green light of the argon laser is absorbed readily by soft tissues, especially when they are pigmented with melanin or haemoglobin. As argon laser energy is converted into heat, there is a thermal effect on soft tissues that first produces coagulation and then vaporization.

> It is not absorbed well by hard tissue and no particular care is needed to protect the teeth during surgery.

Uses:

❖ Argon lasers have an affinity for darker colored tissues and also for hemoglobin, making them excellent coagulators. Thus, an argon laser focused on bleeding vessels stop the hemorrhage.

❖ Argon beam is highly absorbed by hemoglobin, it is an excellent haemostatic laser and can also be used to excise gingival soft tissue lesions.

❖ There is ample evidence that the argon laser is useful in the reduction of pigmented bacteria within the periodontal pocket. **In 1995, Finkbeiner** coined the term laser pocket thermolysis[20] to describe the reduction of pathogens within the periodontal pocket using an argon laser in conjunction with scaling and root planing. The laser tip is inserted into the pocket, extending to the base and moved around the tooth, circumferentially. The pathogens are carbonized, as are the non-adherent plaque deposits and some of the adherent plaque on the root surface as well. Mechanical root instrumentation follows to remove the material from the pocket. This removal leaves a smooth root surface, which is compatible with the healing of the soft tissue inflammatory lesion.

❖ There are reports that this laser is useful in guided tissue regeneration by the de-epithelialzation of the wound margin.

❖ At present, the argon laser is useful in the clinical application of soft tissue welding and soldering. The importance of tissue welding compared with conventional tissue closure methods lies in the fact it can be faster, less traumatic, and easier to apply.

❖ It is effective in the treatment of superficial hemangiomas like port wine stain and removal of some tattoos.

Nd:YAG LASER[21, 79, 86]

➤ It was developed by "**Geusic et al in 1964**".

➤ The first reported use of a fiber-optic–delivered laser in periodontal surgery was the Nd:YAG laser as presented by **Myers et al in 1985.**

➤ With a wavelength of 1064nm, Neodymium:Yttrium-Aluminum-Garnet (Nd:YAG) laser emits light in the near infra-red area of the spectrum.

➤ A flash pump is used as the energy source to activate a Nd:YAG crystal .

➤ This system uses a fiber-optic cable to deliver the light to a conventional hand piece and uses a lens to produce a free beam of laser light.

➤ It shows low absorption with water as well as hydroxyapatite.

➤ Therefore the laser power diffuses deeply through the enamel and dentin and finally heats the pulp.

➤ Thus, they have various degrees of optical scattering and penetration to the tissue, minimal absorption and no reflection.

➤ Nd:YAG lasers work either by a contact or non-contact mode. When working on tissue, however, the contact mode in highly recommended.

➤ As it is also an invisible light so an aiming beam is needed for it.

Uses:

- ❖ This laser can be used with specially designed sapphire or ceramic tips and used as a contact laser scalpel or ablation tool with excellent hemostasis and cutting abilities.

- ❖ Because the laser energy is delivered through a fiber-optic tip, it can be used within the gingival pocket.

- ❖ This laser was first approved by FDA, for use in periodontal pockets. Its used as an adjunct and not as the primary instrument.

- ❖ There is a significant amount of evidence that shows that the Nd:YAG laser wavelength has an affinity for pigmentation; it is this characteristic that makes it especially useful in reducing or eliminating the pigmented bacteria commonly associated with periodontitis.

- ❖ When this bacterial reduction is coupled to the conventional instrumentation of the root to remove hard and soft deposits, more effective decontamination of the diseased pocket can occur, therefore achieving a greater amount of pocket reduction during the conservative phase of periodontal therapy.

- ❖ When used in a contact mode, the Nd:YAG laser is useful in gingivectomy and gingivoplasty procedures. It provides excellent hemostasis and, because the pulsed Nd:YAG laser does not cause deep thermal damage, there is a reduction in postoperative pain.

- ❖ Several Nd:YAG surgical procedures such as a frenectomy may be performed without bleeding and with minimal anesthesia.

- ❖ The Nd:YAg laser is available in continuous wave,pulsed or Q-switched modes and is excellent for the treatment of vascular lesions and intra-oral and extra-oral pigmented lesions and for achieving hemostasis.

- ❖ In addition to excisional and ablative procedures in the oral cavity, the use of the Nd:YAG laser to provide palliative treatment for oral lesions such as aphthous ulcers has been well documented.

49

❖ The laser is used in a noncontact mode at extremely low power to denature the proteins of the surface layer of the lesions, thereby providing a biologic bandage created with the patient's own tissues. This process results in the immediate relief of pain and there is evidence that the healing time may be reduced significantly.

Clinical Sudies:

➢ **Horton & Lin**[39] compared subgingival application of the Nd:YAG laser with conventional scaling and root planing. Each of three segments in 15 patients received Nd:YAG laser irradiation (2 W:100 mJ/pulse and 20 Hz, 2 min), scaling and root planing by curette, or no treatment. The subgingival application with the Nd:YAG laser was equally or more effective than scaling and root planing in reducing or inhibiting recolonization of specific bacterial species and, though less effective in removing calculus, was at least equally effective on measures of probe depths and attachment loss.

➢ **Liu et al**[49] performed a randomized, controlled clinical trial in a split-mouth design, comparing the effects of Nd:YAG laser treatment with scaling and root planing treatment on crevicular IL-1b levels, which is closely associated with periodontal destruction, in 52 sites from eight patients. Data showed that laser therapy alone was less effective than traditional SRP for the reduction of crevicular IL-1b. Laser treatment followed by SRP after 6 weeks showed greater reduction of IL-1b and more clinical improvement than scaling and root planing followed by laser treatment after 6 weeks.

➢ **White et al**[88] recommended 1.5 W (100 mJ/pulse, 15 Hz) irradiation for removal of the sulcular diseased tissue and 2.0 W (100 mJ/pulse, 20 Hz) irradiation for coagulation of soft tissue wall after mechanical debridement.

- **Coluzzi et al[17]** recommended laser soft tissue curettage at 1.8 W (30 mJ/pulse, 60 Hz) after mechanical debridement, followed by irradiation at 2 W (100 mJ/pulse, 20 Hz) for hemostasis and bacterial reduction.

- **Gutknecht et al[35]** suggested the use of the Nd:YAG laser at 2 W (100 mJ/pulse, 20 Hz) for curettage before mechanical debridement to reduce the risk of bacteremia after the scaling and root planing procedures, and to facilitate mechanical debridement.

- **Akira Miyazaki, Toshikazu Yamaguchi et al[2]**, studied the effects of Nd:YAG and carbon dioxide laser treatment and compared it with the ultra-sonic scaling on periodontal pockets of chronic periodontitis patients. They studied 18 patients, each of whom had 2 or more sites with probing depth measuring more than 5mm divided into 3 groups with treatment by Nd : YAG laser alone, or carbon dioxide laser alone or ultra-sonic scaling alone. Their results showed that the Nd:YAG laser shows significant improvement regarding all clinical parameters compared to carbon dioxide and ultra-sonic groups.

- **Mehta.J et al[51]**, carried out a short term assessment of the Nd:YAG Laser With and Without Sodium Fluoride Varnish in the Treatment of Dentin Hypersensitivity. The combination of Nd:YAG laser and 5% sodium fluoride varnish seems to show an impressive efficacy, when compared to either treatment alone, in treating dentin hypersensitivity.

HOL:YAG LASER[20, 21, 86]

- The Holmium:Yttrium-Aluminium-Garnet(Hol:YAG) laser emits light at 2140nm in the infrared region of the spectrum.

- As it is also an invisible light, so a crystal is used as the laser medium as well as the aiming beam. The Hol:YAg laser uses fiberoptic cable to deliver laser energy in the pulsed mode and it can be used in both contact and non contact mode.

- These lasers work well in a water medium and are absorbed well by synovium and joint surfaces.

51

Uses:

➢ Ho:YAG lasers has an affinity for white tissues and is an excellent laser for arthroscopic Temporomandibular Joint Surgery.

➢ It also has the ability to pass through water and is excellent coagulators.

ER:YAG LASER[20, 21, 29, 84, 86]

➢ 1974, **Zharikow et al.**[91]

➢ The Er:YAG is a very promising laser system because the emission wavelength of 2.94 μm coincides with the main absorption peak of water resulting in good absorption in all biological tissues including enamel and dentin.

➢ The FDA approved the pulsed Er:YAG laser for hard tissue treatment such as caries removal and cavity preparation in 1997, for soft tissue surgery and sulcular debridement in 1999 and for osseous surgery in 2004.

➢ The Erbium:Yttrium-Aluminium-Garnet (Er:YAG) laser operates at wavelength of 2940nm via an articulated arm.

➢ The presumed advantage of the Er: YAG laser is its ability to remove superficial skin layers more precisely.

➢ The recently introduced Erbium, Chromium-doped: Yttrium-Scandium-Gallium-Garnet (Er,Cr:YSGG) laser with 2,780 nm wavelength and the Erbium-doped: Yttrium-Scandium-Gallium-Garnet (Er:YSGG) laser with 2,790 nm wavelength, which are more highly absorbed by OH ions than water molecules also have a performance similar to that of the Er:YAG laser.

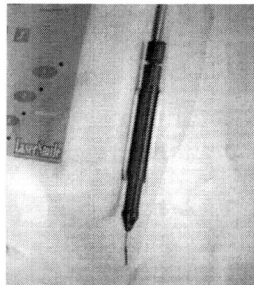

An Er:YAG Delivery Handpiece

Uses:

❖ Recently they are used for the facial resurfacing and incision and ablation of soft tissue.

Microexplosion:

A mechanism of biological tissue ablation with the Er:YAG laser has been proposed by Seka et al[72], in 1996, based on the optical properties of its emission wavelength and morphologic features of the surface ablated by Er:YAG laser. During Er:YAG laser irradiation, the laser energy is absorbed selectively by water molecules and hydrous organic components of biological tissues, causing evaporation of water and organic components and resulting in thermal effects due to the heat generated by this process 'photothermal evaporation'. Moreover, in hard tissue procedures, the water vapor production induces an increase of internal pressure within the tissue, resulting in explosive expansion called 'microexplosion'. These dynamic effects cause mechanical tissue collapse, resulting in a 'thermomechanical' or 'photomechanical' ablation.

❖ Er:YAG can also be used for bone ablation and has indications in soft tissue surgeries where no coagulation effect is desired such as removal of hyperplastic gingival tissue, periodontal surgery and ablation of large benign lesions of the oral mucosa and skin.

❖ As with other soft tissue lasers, there is a proven bactericidal effect when using the Er:YAG laser. Ando et al[4] reported that the Er:YAG laser exhibits a high bactericidal potential against periodontopathic bacteria such as P. gingivalis and Actinobacillus actinomycetemcomitans at a low energy level of 0.3 J/cm2.

❖ **Yamaguchi et al**[89] showed in vitro that the infrared spectrum of bacterial lipopolysaccharide had a peak at 2,940 nm, which also corresponded to the wavelength of the Er:YAG laser, and that the Er:YAG laser at 100 mJ/pulse and 1 Hz (35.4 mJ/cm2) could effectively and rapidly remove most of the lipopolysaccharide that had been coated on the extracted root surfaces.

❖ The most useful application of these lasers in soft tissue surgery occurs when they are used to trim gingival tissues in preparation for caries removal without the need for analgesia.

❖ Research shows that the Er:YAG laser can remove calculus and lipopolysaccharides from root surfaces without melting, charring, or carbonization of the root surface.

❖ The Er:YAG laser may be used not only to remove the diseased hard and soft tissue from root surfaces but also to clean out diseased tissue in root furcations and infrabony pockets without harming root surfaces.

❖ Whereas other wavelengths studied (Nd:YAG, carbon dioxide) may leave a char layer on the root surface that prevents attachment of fibroblasts to the root surface, the Er:YAG leaves a smooth char-free surface, with no smear layer and the collagen matrix exposed.

Clinical Studies:

➢ **Watanabe et al**[83] in 1996 was the first to perform in vivo Er:YAG laser scaling. They reported that the Er:YAG laser could remove calculus from root surfaces in 95% of cases. Although scaled sites showed some irregularity, this was not clinically significant in 98% of cases, and reduction of pocket depth was obtained.

➢ **Schwarz et al**[70] in 1999 reported interesting clinical data of nonsurgical periodontal treatment, comparing Er:YAG laser irradiation with conventional scaling and root planing in a randomized, controlled clinical study using a split-mouth design in 20 patients. At a 6-month post-treatment evaluation, the laser treatment showed similar or better results than the scaling and root planing treatment in terms of reduction of bleeding on probing, pocket depth, and clinical attachment level. In particular, the laser group presented a significantly higher reduction of bleeding on probing and improvement of clinical attachment level compared to the scaling and root planing group. Furthermore, the difference between laser and hand instrumentation in treatment outcomes was much more significant in deeper pockets. The researchers concluded that the Er:YAG laser may present a suitable alternative to conventional mechanical debridement in non surgical periodontal treatment.

➤ **Jurg Eberhard, Heiko Elers et al[43]**, studied the efficacy of subgingival calculus removal with Er:YAG compared to mechanical debridement in 2 groups of 40 teeth each. They found no major difference or statistical significance between periodontally involved root surfaces treated with an Er:YAG laser compared to hand instrumentation.

➤ **Albert Mehl, Reinhardt Wickel et al[3]**, studied the Anti-microbial effects of 2.94 um Er:YAG laser irradiation on the root surfaces of 125 teeth. They reported a significant decrease in anti-microbial levels compared to baseline with a statistical significance of $p<0.05$. They concluded that the Er:YAG had a good potential as a root surface debriding device.

➤ **Sculean et al[71]** in 2004 compared the effectiveness of an Er:YAG laser to that of ultrasonic scaler for non surgical periodontal treatment. Six months following treatment, there was a statistically significant improvement in the mean values of bleeding on probing, probing pocket depth, and clinical attachment level in both groups. However, no statistically or clinically significant differences were observed between the treatment modalities.

➤ **Haim T et al[37]**, saw that the depigmentation of gingival melanin pigmentation by erbium:YAG laser radiation in a defocused mode was a safe and effective procedure. The esthetic results were pleasing and healing was uneventful.

➤

DIODE LASERS[16]

> The diode laser is a solid-state semiconductor laser that typically uses a combination of Gallium (Ga), Arsenide (Ar), and other elements such as Aluminum (Al) and Indium (In) to change electrical energy into light energy.

> This "chip" of material has the optical resonator mirrors directly attached to its ends, and an electrical current is used as the pumping mechanism.

> The wavelength range is about 800– 980 nm. The available wavelengths for dental use range from about 800 nm for the active medium containing aluminium to 980 nm for the active medium composed of indium.

> The laser is emitted in continuous-wave and gated-pulsed modes, and is usually operated in a contact method using a flexible fiber optic delivery system.

> Laser light at 800–980 nm is poorly absorbed in water, but highly absorbed in hemoglobin and other pigments.

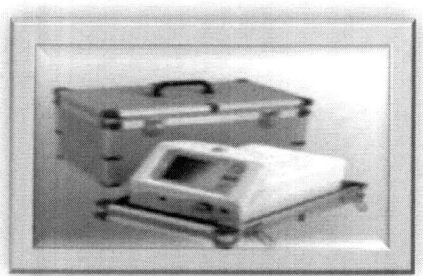

> Since the diode basically does not interact with dental hard tissues, the laser is an excellent soft tissue surgical laser, indicated for cutting and coagulating gingiva and oral mucosa, and for soft tissue curettage or sulcular debridement.

- The FDA approved oral soft tissue surgery in 1995 and sulcular debridement in 1998 by means of a diode laser (GaAlAs 810 nm).
- The diode laser exhibits thermal effects using the 'hot-tip' effect caused by heat accumulation at the end of the fiber, and produces a relatively thick coagulation layer on the treated surface. The usage is quite similar to electrocauterization.
- The advantages of diode lasers are the smaller size of the units as well as the lower financial costs.

Uses:

- Used for all soft tissue procedures performed by Nd:YAG & carbon dioxide lasers.
- The affinity of the diode laser wavelength (819nm) for anaerobic pathogens may be a useful method for decontaminating the surface of failing implants in peri-implantitis.
- **Moritz et al,** saw considerable bacterial elimination from periodontal pockets at a much higher level than scaling group alone, when using diode lasers.
- There is evidence that this wavelength may cause a reduction in gingival inflammation and a reduced need for local anesthetic during surgical procedures.
- The laser may be used in a noncontact mode to coagulate soft tissues or to provide hemostasis over an area.
- In addition to soft tissue surgeries, a diode laser may be used to identify and quantify the degree of caries.
- Low-level laser therapy is provided by semiconductor instruments emitting visible and invisible near infrared light energy at powers significantly below any surgical interactive threshold. They can provide biostimulation and pain relief.

Clinical Studies:

- ➤ **Moritz et al**[55, 56] reported pocket irradiation with a diode laser (805 nm) following scaling. Irradiation with the diode laser, produced considerable bacterial elimination from periodontal pockets at a much higher level than the scaling alone group, especially in terms of A. actinomycetemcomitans. They concluded that diode laser therapy, in combination with scaling, supports healing of periodontal pockets by eliminating bacteria.

- ➤ **Coluzzi**[17] recommended laser soft tissue curettage at 0.4 W in continuous wave mode after mechanical debridement of root surface, followed by irradiation at 0.6 W for hemostasis and bacterial reduction.

- ➤ **Gutknecht et al** suggested the use of a diode laser at continuous wave mode for curettage before mechanical debridement.

- ➤ Further detailed studies are required to establish proper irradiation conditions, including the use of water coolant, for periodontal pocket therapy with diode lasers.

KTP LASER[20, 21, 86]

- ➤ This is a modified version of Nd: YAG laser.

- ➤ With the frequency-double quenching crystal, this laser emits laser light at the 532-nm wavelength, or half the wavelength of the Nd:YAG.

- ➤ This system usually utilizes a fiberoptic cable with a handpiece.

- ➤ Absorption is similar to that of the argon laser and has been used in the treatment of argon laser

Uses:

KTP lasers are uses in the treatment of:-

- ❖ Vascular and pigmented lesions,

- ❖ Tattoo removal

❖ Blepharoplasty etc.

Q-SWITCHED RUBY LASER[20, 21, 86]

➢ Q-Switched ruby laser produces visible, pulsed red light at 694-nm wavelength.

➢ This red light is absorbed by melanin, green and blue black pigments.

➢ Pulse width as small as 20 nanoseconds can be achieved by the currently available systems. Fiberoptics can be utilized with handpiece to treat some pigmented lesions and tattoos effectively.

Uses:

❖ This laser is very effective in removing pigmented lesions, blue and black tattoos with minimal scarring.

FLASH LAMP-PUMPED PULSED DYE (FLPPD) LASER[9, 21]

➢ This laser produces yellow visible light in the 400- to 1000-nm range and is most commonly tuned at 510:577, or 585nm.

➢ This specific wavelength is determined by the dye chosen and can be used for the specific tissue to be removed, offering great flexibility.

Uses:

This versatile laser is used in treatment of:-

❖ Pigmented and hemopigmented lesions,

❖ Scar removal,

❖ Achieving hemostasis,

❖ Photodynamic cancer therapy,

❖ Ablation of salivary gland ,

❖ Kidney stones removal

❖ Tattoo removal.

COPPER VAPOR LASER[21]

➢ These lasers work at the wavelength of 511 and 578 nm, and are similar to both the KTP and argon lasers.

➢ Its medium used for this is highly heated copper producing gas.

➢ The light produced by the reaction with this medium is delivered down a fiberoptic cable in the pulsed mode.

Uses:

❖ It is effective in the treatment of hemorrhagic telengectasias and it has also been used to ablate some pigmented lesions.

EXCIMER LASER[21]

➢ These lasers emit ultraviolet light at 193 to 351nm, using halide gases for a medium. In this system electrical current charges halide gases to excite photons.

➢ These lasers used fiber-optic cable to deliver pulsed laser energy.

➢ It acts through photochemical effect by breaking the organic molecule bonds i.e. ionization at a microscopic scale, hence electron detachment.

➢ It generates neither heat nor optical breakdown.

➢ Among the 20 or so excimer molecules investigated, two wavelengths (193nm and 308nm) allow preparation without heating.

➢ It appears that the Argon fluoride excimer laser allows preparation without heating.

- The ablation depth per pulse in healthy enamel amounts to 0.15μm and in healthy dentin to 0.20μm in a 1mm2 focus area with an energy density of about 10mJ/cm2 pulse.

Uses:

- These are used for keratotomy to reshape corneal tissue and correct poor vision.

ALEXANDRITE LASER[21]

- This Q-Switched laser produces red light of the 755nm from a crystal of Alexandrite and uses a flexible waveguide.
- It is well absorbed by green, black, and dark blue pigments.
- The long wavelength of the laser allows deeper penetration.

Uses:

- Used for the treatment of pigmented lesions that extend deeper into the dermal layer.
- Lightening of congenital nevi.
- The Q-switching mechanism produces a high intensity pulse of 50 to 100 nanosecond that can be used effectively in the removal of tattoos with blue, green and black pigments.
- Under water cooling, selectively ablates supra & sub gingival calculus as well as dental plaque.

ADVANTAGES OF LASERS [29, 50, 85]

- Hemostasis
- Precise cutting of the tissues
- Minimal disturbance of the surrounding tissues
- Prevention of tumor seeding.
- Reduces surgical time

- ➢ Reduced post operative pain.

- ➢ Reduced post operative edema

- ➢ Bacterial reduction

- ➢ Sterilization of wound

- ➢ Microscopic & endoscopic control

- ➢ Better patient co-operation

- ➢ Flexibility

- ➢ Fast productivity

- ➢ No drilling noise

- ➢ No vibration

- ➢ Increased bond strength of white fillings to tooth

- ➢ Reduced sensitivity after filling

- ➢ Immediate cosmetic results possible

DISADVANTAGES OF LASERS[20, 25, 61]

- ➢ Costly armamentarium

- ➢ Technique sensitive

- ➢ Thoroughly trained & high skilled professional required

- ➢ Harmful effects to eyes

- ➢ Harmful effects to skin

- ➢ Multiple laser could be required for treatment

- ➢ Local infection could complicate laser treatment

- ➢ Scarring or altered skin texture is also a possibility

POTENTIAL HAZARDS OF LASERS[20, 25, 61]

Safety is an integral part of the dental treatment with a laser instrument. Lasers are classified according to the potential hazards is based on the potential of the primary laser beam or reflected beam to cause biologic damage to eyes & skin[21]. These lasers can lead to various effects such as ocular injury, tissue damage, respiratory hazards etc.

According to ANSI standard Z136.1-2000, Occupational Safety and Health Administration (OSHA) & American Conference of Governmental Industrial Hygienists in 2004, classified lasers according to the output power of continuous emission lasers or energy per pulse for pulsed lasers and amount of time the beam is viewed.

The higher the classification number, greater is the potential hazard[61].

Class I: Device is completely enclosed. Do not pose any health hazard.

Class II: Emit only visible light with low power output. Do not normally pose a hazard because of normal blinking & aversion reactions.

Class II a: Hazardous when directly viewed for longer than 1000 seconds

Class II b: Hazardous when there is viewing time of more than one fourth of a second is there.

Class III a: These laser can emit any wavelength and have output power of 0.5 W of visible light. When viewed momentarily it will not harm the patient. These lasers come with a caution label on it.

Class III b: Can produce hazard if viewed directly or viewed from reflected light for any duration.

Class IV: Any output greater than 0.5 W measured in either the continuous wave or pulsed emission constitutes class IV. They are hazardous from direct viewing and may produce hazardous diffuse reflections.

According to British Standard BS 4803[86] it was classified as:-

Classification according to potential hazards[61, 85]		
Class	Risk	Examples
I	Fully enclosed system	Nd:YAG welding laser system used in dental laboratory
II	Visible low power laser protected by the blink reflex	Visible red aiming beam of a surgical laser.
IIIa	Visible laser above 1 milliwatt	No dental examples
IIIb	Higher power laser unit (up to 0.5 watts) which may or may not be visible .direct viewing hazardous to the eyes	Low power Diode (50 milliwatt) laser used for bio stimulation.
IV	Damage to eyes & skin possible .Direct Or Indirect Viewing Hazardous To The Eyes.	All lasers used for oral surgery, whitening and cavity preparation.

PREVENTIVE MEASURES[61]:

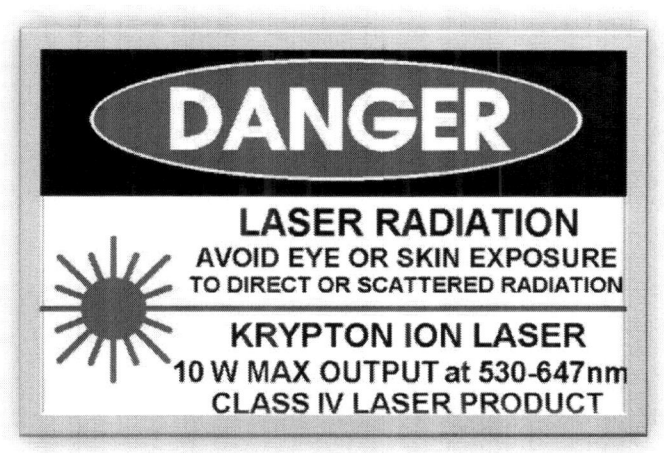

Warning Sign During Laser Application

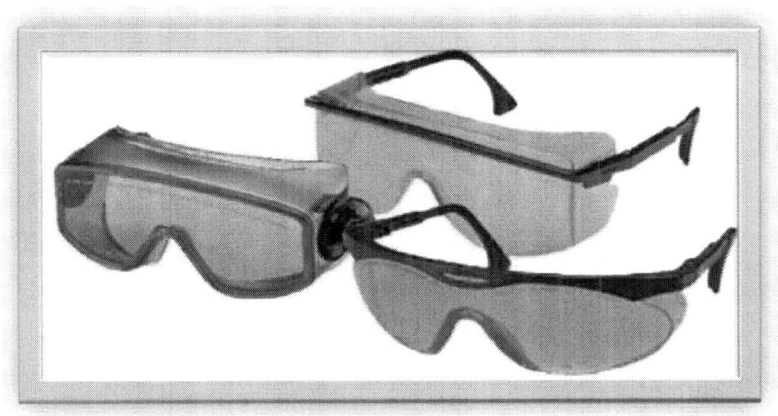

Protective Eye Gear

In the clinical practice the following protective measures taken to avoid the various hazardous effects of lasers. These are:

For the hazardous effects of lasers on clinician & patient:

- Proper time & power setting to be maintained
- Use of eye glasses specific for each wavelength
- Proper ventilation,
- High volume suction,
- Masks filters face masks,
- Shield & Cap

For the fire and explosion hazards:

- Use only wet or fire retardant material in the operative field
- Use only non-combustible anesthetic agents
- Avoid alcohol based topical anesthetic
- Avoid alcohol moistened gauze while firing the laser.
- Protect tissue adjacent to surgical site.
- Know operation & location of nearest fire extinguisher.
- Store safely all the combustible material outside the hazardous zone.
- According to ANSI standard Z136.1-2000 Guidelines "Nitrous Oxide supports combustion & should not be used during laser surgery.

CLINICAL APPLICATIONS

According to **Convissor. R.A (2004)**[19], Lasers have various clinical applications in dentistry. These are:-

1. CLINICAL APPLICATIONS IN ORAL MEDICINE/ORAL PATHOLOGY/ORAL SURGERY

➢ Biopsy

➢ Operculectomy

➢ Apicoectomy

➢ Oral soft tissue lesions

➢ Treatment of aphthous ulcers

➢ Treatment of cold sores/ herpes – early intervention can prevent sore from developing

2. CLINICAL APPLICATIONS IN PERIODONTICS

➢ Initial pocket therapy

➢ Non osseous gingival surgery

➢ Frenectomy

➢ Gingivectomy

➢ Graft

➢ De – epethelialization

➢ Removal of granulomatous tissue

➢ Osseous recontouring

3. CLINICAL APPLICATIONS IN PROSTHODONTICS

A. Removable Prosthodontics:

➢ Epulis fissuratum

➢ Denture stomatitis

> Residual ridge modification

> Tuberosity reduction

> Torus reduction

> Soft tissue modification

B. Fixed Prosthodontics/Cosmetics:

> Crown lengthening

> Osseous crown lengthening

> Formation of ovate pontic sites

> Altered passive eruption management

> Modification of soft tissue around laminates

> Bleaching

C. Implantology:

> Second-stage recovery

> Peri-implantitis

4. CLINICAL APPLICATIONS IN ORTHODONTICS/ PEDODONTICS

> Exposure of teeth

> Soft tissue management of orthodontic patients

5. CLINICAL APPLICATIONS IN OPERATIVE DENTISTRY

> Deciduous teeth treatment

> Permanent teeth treatment

Whenever a new surgical device enters the arena, there is always skepticism, hesitation, caution, and rejection. It should be emphasized that lasers are only an alternative to conventional surgical systems. When used correctly in proven applications, lasers offer an acceptable and impressive alternative within the field of Periodontics and in other related dental fields.

LASER PERIOTHERAPY

Lasers were first employed in dentistry in hard tissue treatments, such as caries removal and cavity preparation, as a substitute for mechanical cutting and drilling. After the discovery of the ruby laser in 1960, **Goldman and coworkers** attempted caries removal in vitro using the ruby laser in 1964. Since then, many researchers have investigated the effects of various lasers such as the argon, carbon dioxide, and Nd:YAG lasers on dental hard tissues and caries. However, previous laser systems were basically not indicated for hard tissue procedures due to major thermal damage. Thus, these laser systems showed only limited potential for caries prevention and for the polymerization of light-cured restorative materials in the field of preventive and operative dentistry. The real revolution in laser therapy came in the late 1990's when FDA approval was given for soft tissue applications like sulcular debridement, gingivoplasty and frenectomies. This lead to the immediate use of soft tissue lasers in myriad ways by periodontists, limited only by the power of their ingenuity.

There are several advantages to using lasers in periodontal therapy. These advantages include hemostasis, less postoperative swelling, a reduction in bacterial population at the surgical site, less need for suturing, faster healing, and less postoperative pain. Studies on the speed of healing of laser wounds compared with scalpel wounds presently are inconclusive: several studies suggest faster healing, some suggest slower healing, and still others report that there is no difference.

NON SURGICAL THERAPY WITH LASERS

The initial and most important stage of periodontal therapy is the non surgical mechanical debridement of periodontally diseased root surfaces.

Since the periodontium is composed of gingiva, periodontal ligament, cementum, and alveolar bone, both soft and hard tissues are always targeted when using lasers for the treatment of periodontal lesions. The commonly used high power lasers, carbon dioxide and Nd:YAG are capable of excellent soft tissue ablation, and have an adequate hemostatic effect. As such, these lasers have been generally approved for soft tissue management in periodontics and oral surgery. However, these lasers are not useful for the treatment of the root surface or alveolar bone, due to carbonization of these tissues and major thermal side-effects on the target and surrounding tissues. In 1989, **Keller, Hibst and Kayano et al[46]**, reported the possibility of dental hard tissue ablation by Er:YAG laser irradiation, which is highly absorbed by water. In 2004**, Aoki et al[5]** reported that Er:YAG laser is capable of removing sub gingival calculus without a major change of the root surface. Frequency-doubled Alexandrite laser is able to remove supra & sub gingival calculus as well as dental plaque in a completely selective manner without ablating the underlying enamel & cementum, as reported by **Rechmann in 2004.**

Conventional methods are not completely effective in eliminating all types of bacteria. There has been a shift in emphasis, from a purely mechanical approach to the use of novel technical modalities having additional bactericidal effects, such as lasers. The ideal properties of a wavelength that can be used successfully for a non-surgical periodontal therapy are bactericidal, easy to deliver into the pocket, and safe enough to use in a periodontal pocket so that it causes no harm to the root surface. In a study conducted by Moritz et al, using diode lasers, the investigators concluded that the diode lasers revealed a bactericidal effect, helped reduce inflammation, and supported the healing of periodontal pockets through the elimination of bacteria. Nd:YAG laser is capable of eliminating endotoxins, as was shown by White in 1991. Following the application of Nd:YAG alone there is a decrease in Pg, decrease in volume of GCF & interleukin-1 in GCF samples, as was shown by **Miyazaki et al, 2003.**

Carbon dioxide laser in a defocusing mode has bactericidal effects. Er:YAG laser has bactericidal effect. It removes toxins diffused into root cementum, such as bacterial LPS. Argon laser is effective in clinical infections caused by biofilm-associated Species; eg. Prevotella & Porphyromonas.

Bader[7] described the advantage of laser curettage as enhanced bacterial reduction with good hemostasis. He concluded that when laser energy is directed parallel to the root surface, the laser removes the bacteria and endotoxins from the soft tissues. If the laser energy is directed onto the root surface rather than the soft tissue lining of the periodontal pocket, the root surface can be damaged. **Schwarz et al[69]** studied the effects of a diode laser on the root surface and they concluded that when the laser energy is directed onto the root surface, severe damage, including crater like defects and grooves, occurred on the root surface. **Morlock et al[57]** found similar results with Nd:YAG lasers. **Schwartz in 2001,**showed a decrease in bleeding on probing and probing depth; and an increase in clinical attachment level, when using the Er:YAG laser.

Thus, lasers are used as an adjunct to standard treatments rather than as a replacement for standard treatments. Laser curettage of periodontal pockets is unsuccessful unless combined with standard scaling and root planning to remove bacteria and accretions from the root surface. **Neil and Mellonig[60]** and **Moritz et al[55, 56];** emphasized in their clinical studies that the most significant improvement was found in the group of patients who had conventional scaling combined with laser treatment. Conventional instruments are used for standard scaling and root planning procedures and lasers are used solely for the soft tissue lining the pocket wall. The conclusion to be reached from this is that the diode and Nd:YAg lasers are effective wavelengths to be used in non-surgical periodontal therapy, when used according to the established protocols.

SURGICAL LASER THERAPY

The development of lasers as a modality of therapy in the management of periodontal lesions and conditions is an ongoing and exciting discipline. No area of dentistry has seen more changes with laser therapy than the field of Periodontics. The development of the laser therapy for soft tissue manipulation has been progressing rather more rapidly than its use as an adjunct in the management of the infectious aspect of Periodontitis. One of the first carbon dioxide lasers used for soft tissue applications in Periodontics was introduced in 1987 by **Pick et al.** Although carbon dioxide lasers were generally used in non-contact mode, the newer hollow wave guide delivery systems allow for focused delivery of the energy to within 0.1mmof the target tissue in a Cutting Mode. Erbium, Holmium, and Excimer lasers have been used for osseous surgical and soft tissue sculpting procedures. Lasers today are becoming portable and are being used for an ever-increasing variety of periodontal soft tissue applications.

For a periodontal surgical procedure to be successful with optimal tissue regeneration, complete debridement and decontamination of root surface and bone defect is necessary. Laser application is effective in debriding areas of limited accessibility, such as deep intrabony defects & furcation areas where mechanical instruments cannot eliminate microbiological etiologic factors. The Nd;YAG and diode lasers have shown a great deal of success in treating molars with furcation involvements and Class-II mobility.

Whatever wavelength is used for regenerative periodontal surgery must not cause any harmful effects on the root surfaces. **Trylovich et al**[81] evaluated the effects of Nd:YAG laser of fibroblast attachment to endotoxin -treated root surfaces. These investigators concluded that lasers alter the cementum surface in a way that they make it unfavourable for fibroblast attachment. **Spencer et al**[75], **Thomas et al**[50] **and others**[42, 66] also found that when the Nd:YAG laser is used directly on the root surface, the surface is altered unfavourably. **Schwarz et al**[69] in a study compared a diode laser, an Er:YAG laser and scaling and root planning. He concluded that the Er:YAG treatment left the root surfaces smooth, with no cracks or thermal effects. One of the most significant studies detailing the potential for the use of Er:YAG lasers for periodontal regeneration was performed again by **Schwarz et al**[70]. They studied the in vivo effects of the Er:YAG laser on the biocompatibility of the periodontally diseased root surfaces and periodontal ligament fibroblasts. Their results showed that the Er:YAG laser promotes the attachment of the periodontal ligament fibroblasts on previously diseased root surfaces and the surface structure of the Er:YAG laser instrumented roots offers better conditions for the adherence of periodontal fibroblasts than scaling and root planing.

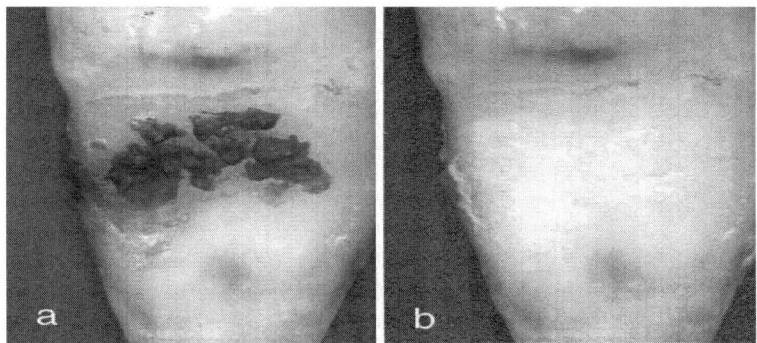

Photographs of the root surfaces before and after ER:YAG laser scaling of subgingival calculus

There is a great deal of difference between the use of Er:YAG laser(2790nm) and the Er:Cr:YSGG laser(2940 nm) in regenerative surgical periodontics. The American Academy of Periodontology has stated that the Er:YAG laser offers the best application of laser use directly on the hard tissue, leaving the least thermal damage and creating a surface that suggests biocompatibility for soft tissue attachment. Studies have shown the ability of the Er:YAG laser to remove lipopolysaccharides from the root surfaces, facilitate the removal of the smear layer after root planning, remove calculus and cementum[66]. The Er:YAG laser is an excellent choice to use in regenerative periodontal surgery to prepare the root surface for new attachment of connective tissue. The problem lies in ensuring that the connective tissue rather than the epithelium has an opportunity to grow and create new attachment.

73

DE-EPITHELISATION:

The successful treatment of periodontal defects requires new attachment of the periodontal ligament fibres into the newly forming cementum of the root surface. Apical proliferation of epithelium from the adjacent surfaces of the wound along a healing surface interferes with the formation of a new connective attachment between the root surface and the supporting alveolar bone. Many techniques have been suggested to retard the downward growth of epithelium.

Various types of materials have been placed between the edge of the healing wound and the root surface in an attempt to retard epithelial migration. Until the advent of resorbable barrier membranes that would maintain their integrity for a long enough period of time for attachment to occur, a method of epithelial exclusion using a carbon dioxide laser was suggested.

Rossman et al[67] used monkeys to determine the ability of the carbon dioxide laser to prevent epithelial migration after flap surgery. The results showed that the epithelisation of the carbon dioxide treated side was delayed by atleast 7 days, allowing for new connective tissue to grow. The investigators concluded that the carbon dioxide laser can be used to delay the apical down growth of the epithelium and that this technique was technically less demanding and more time efficient than the other currently known methods of epithelial retardation. **Israel et al**[40] used the carbon dioxide laser in a human study and showed that the non-lased teeth healed with a long junctional epithelium whereas the notch in the lased teeth showed connective tissue and some repair cementum. The in vivo human results showed that the carbon dioxide laser de-epithelisation technique has the abiity to obtain new clinical attachment with bone fill in previously diseased sites. Thus, these studies have shown that the carbon dioxide laser can remove epithelium effectively from gingival tissues without damaging the underlying connective tissue.

When sites treated by laser de-epithelialization combined with osseous grafts are compared with nonlased sites in split-mouth experimental designs, the carbon dioxide sites show better gain of clinical attachment level and increased osseous fill of infrabony defects.

The results of the carbon dioxide de-epithelisation studies combined with the Er:YAG studies of the effects on root surfaces lead to the conclusion that the most effective method of regenerative periodontal surgical procedures would be a double-wavelength technique. This technique would use the Er:YAG laser to debride the open surgical site, clean and sterilize the root surface, and prepare the root surface for the adhesion of fibroblasts. The carbon dioxide laser would remove the epithelium, which would allow the fibroblasts to adhere and proliferate, creating new attachment. This double wavelength technique shows tremendous promise in the field of regenerative periodontal surgery[19].

OSSEOUS SURGERY:

Many full-thickness mucoperiosteal flap procedures include osseous resection. The only wavelengths cleared by the FDA for osseous surgery are the erbium family of lasers. The Er:YAG and the Er:Cr:YSGG are the only wavelengths that have the ability to ablate osseous tissue safety[19]. Romano investigated the Er:YAG laser and its ability to cut bone and found that the depth of ablation was linearly related to the number of pulses and that moisture of the surgical site with water spray prevented char formation. It is essential to keep a continuous water spray on the surgical site to act as a heat sink and to keep the energy as low as possible to avoid iatrogenic damage.

Walsh in an early study looked at the role of the erbium lasers in implants, bone, and soft tissue surgery. Sasaki et al looked at the nature of the tissue after irradiation with the Er:YAG wavelength compared with the carbon dioxide laser and bur drilling. Under scanning elevtron microscopy and transmission electron microscopy, they demonstrated that laser irradiation of bone resulted in a changed layer of 30μm thickness, which consisted of two distinct sublayers: a superficial, greatly altered layer and a deeper, less affected layer. They found that the major changes on bone consisted of microcracking, disorganization, slight recrystallisation of the original apatite, and slight reduction of the surrounding organic matter. **Eversole et al** concluded in their article that the Er:Cr;YSGG laser was an effective tool for precise osseous surgery and healing. They concluded that the wound cavities were smooth, clean and straight.

FRENECTOMY[13]:

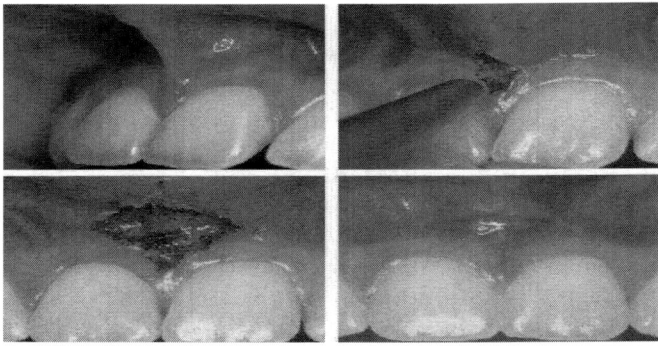

Perhaps one of the most dramatic applications of lasers in periodontics is in frenectomies. The traditional surgical frenectomy uses profound anaesthesia, scalpel and sutures. There usually is a considerable amount of hemorrhage and the post-operative period is quite uncomfortable. A laser frenectomy is bloodless and requires minimal anaesthesia and the char layer left over the ablated frenum allows for little or no discomfort . A few studies have reported delayed wound healing , but the lack of post-operative pain more than compensates for the delayed wound healing. This technique is particularly useful in younger patients as it is more benign compared with the traditional approach.

GINGIVECTOMY AND GINGIVOPLASTY[13]:

Various laser wavelengths can be used for the treatment of gingival enlargements; that are usually the result of intake of certain drugs like calcium-channel blockers and phenytoin, etc. These include carbon dioxide lasers, Er:YAG lasers, Nd:YAG lasers, Diode lasers etc. These lasers can also be used to restore the normal gingival contours.

When using the carbon dioxide laser, a periosteal elevator is placed between the tissue and the tooth, to protect the hard tissue from the effects of the carbon dioxide wavelength. A biologic bandage (char layer) is placed over the surgical site, eliminating the need for a periodontal dressing.

The primary disadvantage of using an Er:YAG laser for soft tissue applications is minimal hemostasis compared with other wavelengths, which could lead to mild bleeding or oozing before hemostasis is achieved. Postoperative recovery usually is uneventful, with little discomfort. Healing is comparable to scalpel incisions.

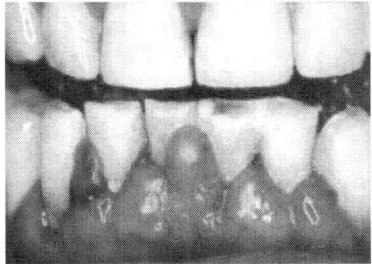

A preoperative view of gingival enlargement caused by a calcium channel blocker

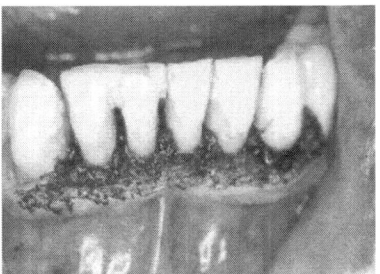

Immediate postoperative photo of the completed gingivectomy

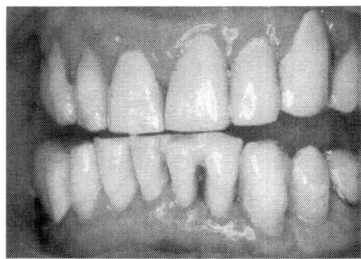

A 4-week postoperative view showing normal gingival contours restored

SOFT TISSUE CROWN LENGTHENING[13]:

Soft tissue crown lengthening can be accomplished easily with a laser when two conditions exist. First, there must be no need to contour the underlying bone; second, there must be sufficient attached gingiva so that there will be an adequate zone of attached gingiva after the soft tissue has been ablated.

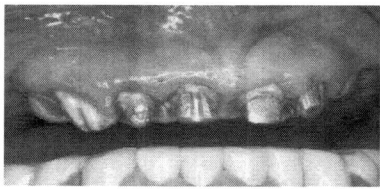

Preoperative view of the surgical site

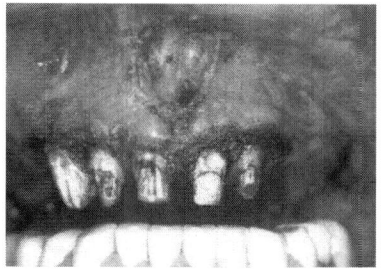

Immediate postoperative view

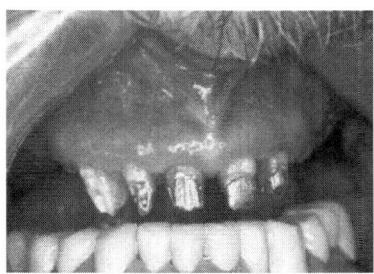

One-month postoperative view

DE-PIGMENTATION[13]:

For depigmentation, Er:YAG is preferred in areas with thin gingival. A carbon dioxide laser when used at 4 W continuous wave in a defocused mode; can separate the epithelium from the underlying connective tissue by creating a blister. Because the melanocytes are found in the basement membrane of the epithelium, they will be permanently eliminated with the tissue that is removed.

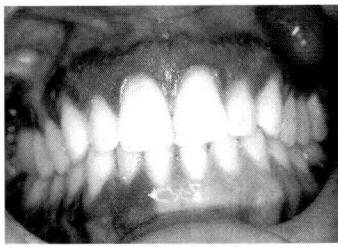

A preoperative view of severe oral pigmentation that is to be removed using a laser peel

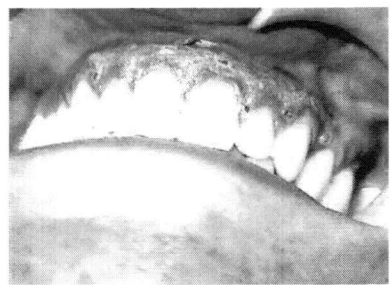

Blister has formed over entire surgical site

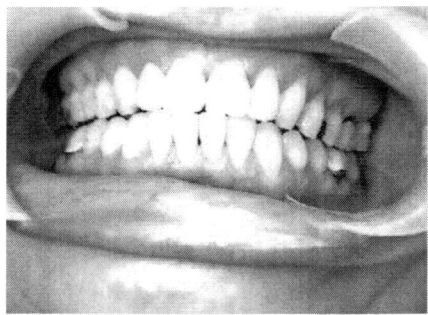

A 16-day postoperative view

FREE GINGIVAL GRAFT[13]:

When placing free gingival grafts, lasers may be used for performing vestibuloplasty. This is done by by placing the laser tip parallel to the mandible in a focused mode and separating the vestibular tissue, leaving the periosteum attached to the bone. At the donor site, lasers can be used to create a biological bandage.

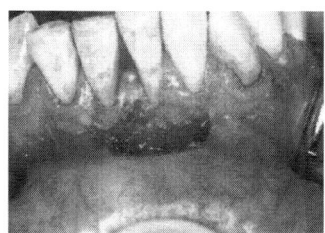

To prepare the recipient site, a vestibuloplasty has been performed using a carbon dioxide laser

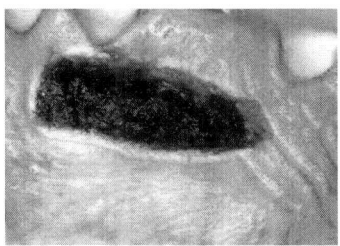

Donor site covered by biologic bandage

LASERS IN DENTAL IMPLANTOLOGY[50]

The advantages of using lasers in implant dentistry are the same as for any other soft tissue dental procedure. These advantages include increased hemostasis, minimal damage to the surrounding tissue, reduced swelling, reduced infection, and reduced pain postoperatively. Due to the hemostasis provided by lasers, there is the significant advantage of improved visibility during surgery. The increasing popularity of the erbium family of lasers, with their hard tissue ablation capability, has added the potential for its use for osteotomy and decontamination of infected and ailing implant bodies.

In the past, controversy has surrounded the use of lasers on dental implants. Each specific wavelength has its own absorption characteristics. As such, although Nd:YAG has been a particularly popular wavelength to use for soft tissue second stage surgery, several investigators contend that it is contraindicated. Walsh, Block et al, and Chu et al studied the effects of this wavelength on implants. The specific issues that were studied were the transmission of heat to the bone from the heated implant surface, effects of this wavelength on the metal surface, the potential for pitting and melting, and the porosity of the implant surface.

Carbon dioxide laser energy, on the other hand, is reflected away from metal surfaces. The failure of implants to absorb the energy of the carbon dioxide laser is a major advantage of this wavelength. Use of the carbon dioxide wavelength minimizes the risk of temperature induced tissue damage as a result of lasing the implant surface. It generally is accepted that the threshold for bone cells to remain viable is a temperature increase from 37°C (normal body temperature) to 47°C. An article by **Mouhyi et al**[59] demonstrated that a carbon dioxide laser on a wet implant surface in pulsed mode at 8W(10 milliseconds pulse duration, 20 Hz for 5 seconds) induced a temperature increase of less than 3°C, well within the 10°C safety margin from 37°C to 47°C. It also should be noted that the hemostatic properties of carbon dioxide are excellent, which is a tremendous advantage for its use on soft tissue.

The erbium family of lasers is similar to the carbon dioxide wavelength in some respects. There is minimal depth of penetration in soft tissue and reflection away from the implant surface. The erbium lasers do not have as significant a hemostatic capability as carbon dioxide or Nd:YAG.

All types of lasers can be used to excise or vaporize periodontal tissue as needed to expose dental implants. One advantage of the use of lasers in implantology is that impressions can be taken immediately after second stage surgery because there is little blood contamination in the field due to the hemostatic effect of the lasers.

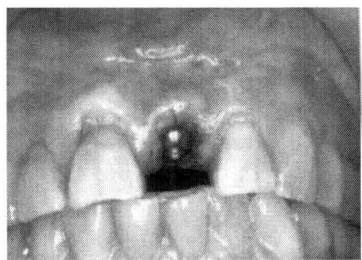

The head of the implant fixture has been exposed using a carbon dioxide laser

There also is minimal tissue shrinkage after laser surgery, which assures that the tissue margins will remain at the same level after healing as they are immediately after the surgery. In addition, the use of the laser can eliminate the trauma to the tissue of flap reflection and suture placement (assuming adequate zones of keratinized tissue and the knowledge of where the implant has been placed).

One of the main reasons dentists cite for using lasers during implant recovery is that there is less postoperative pain, less bleeding, and faster healing; however, there also is the potential for obliteration of the attached gingiva if this technology is overused.

One of the most interesting uses of lasers in implant dentistry is the possibility of salvaging ailing implants by decontaminating their surfaces with laser energy.

Diode lasers were used in a study by **Bach et al**[6] who found a significant improvement in the 5-year survival rate when integrating laser decontamination into the approved treatment protocol. **Dortbudak et al**[24] found that the use of low level laser therapy with a diode soft laser (690 nm) for 60 seconds after the placement of toluidine blue O for 1 minute on the contaminated surface reduced the counts of bacteria by a minimum of 92%.The same group was able to obtain complete bacterial elimination in a study using the 905-nm diode (also a soft tissue laser) with toluidine blue O on all types of implant surfaces. Their data on several implant surfaces suggest that lethal photosensitization, through the use of toluidine blue O to sensitize the cell membranes to laser light, may have potential in the treatment of peri-implantitis.

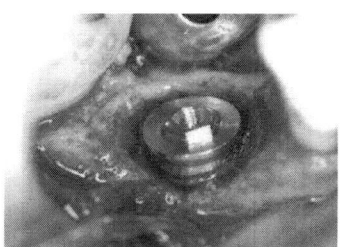

Granulation tissue and exudate around implant fixture

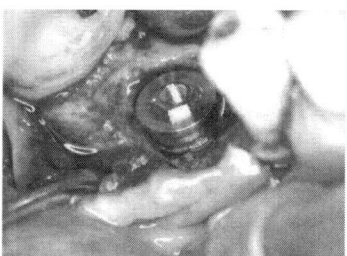

All inflammation removed with diode laser

Carbon dioxide lasers have been successful in decontaminating implant surfaces. **Kato et al**[45] found that this wavelength did not cause surface alteration, rise of temperature, or serious damage of connective tissue cells located outside the irradiation spot or cause inhibition of cell adhesion to the irradiated area. **Mouhyi et al**[58] found that a combination of citric acid, hydrogen peroxide, and carbon dioxide laser irradiation seems to be effective for cleaning and re-establishing the oxide structure of contaminated titanium surfaces. **Romanos**[65] was able to treat successfully 18 ailing implants in 14 patients using mechanical debridement followed by implant surface decontamination with the carbon dioxide laser and subsequent grafting of the bony defects with a resorbable barrier.

The Er:YAG laser also has been proposed for surface decontamination of dental implants. In an article by **Schwarz et al**[68], this wavelength was found to be effective in removing subgingival calculus from titanium implants without leading to any thermal damage.

The previous articles are contrasted with the findings in a study by **Kreisler et al**[48]. They used various wavelengths including Nd:YAG, holmium:yttrium aluminum garnet (Ho:YAG), Er:YAG, carbon dioxide, and gallium-aluminum-arsenide for implant surface decontamination. They concluded that Nd:YAG and Ho:YAG lasers are not suitable for decontamination of dental implant surfaces at any power output. With Er:YAG and carbon dioxide, the power output must be limited so as to avoid surface damage. The gallium-aluminum arsenide laser seems to not cause any surface alterations.

One of the hallmarks of the osseointegration technique is a passive fit of the prosthesis on the implants. It has been proposed that one of the ways to obtain a true passive fit is by the elimination of the casting technique. The expansion and contraction during casting can lead to a nonpassive fit of the implant prosthesis when placed onto multiple implants. To that end, the proposed laser welding of titanium components has been advocated and used with some mixed success.

LOW LEVEL LASER THERAPY[78]

Therapeutic laser treatment, also referred to as low-level laser therapy (LLLT), offers numerous benefits. Along with the primary benefit of being nonsurgical, it promotes tissue healing and reduces edema, inflammation, and pain.

No true side effects of using the low-level laser light have been found. It is noninvasive, nonpharmaceutical, and economical. The principle of using LLLT is to supply direct biostimulative light energy to the body's cells. Cellular photoreceptors can absorb low-level laser light and pass it on to mitochondria, which promptly produce the cell's fuel, ATP.

The mechanisms of action underlying the analgesic effects remain unclear, despite the implicit treatment benefits. There is evidence suggesting that LLLT may have significant neuropharmacologic effects on the synthesis, release, and metabolism of a range of neurochemicals, including serotonin and acetylcholine at the central level and histamine and prostaglandin at the peripheral level. The pain influence has also been explained by the LLLT effect on enhanced synthesis of endorphin, decreased c-fiber activity, bradykinin, and altered pain threshold.

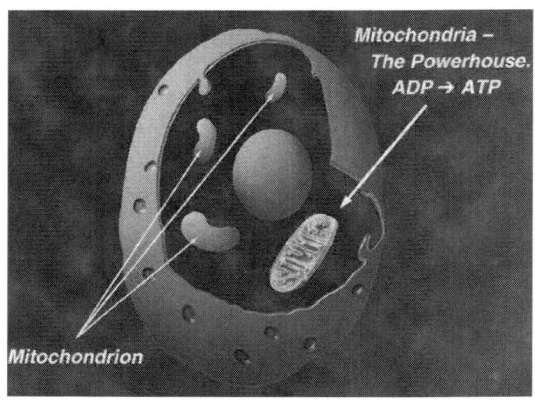

ADP producing ATP

The effect of therapeutic laser irradiation is most prominent in cells in a reduced redox state. This means that the effect on healthy cells is less prominent and transient. Nevertheless, some investigators recommend irradiation before and after surgical interventions. The effect of the laser is localized at the treatment site but can have a more generalized systemic effect. Infrared lasers have greater penetration than lasers in the visible range and are therefore able to affect deeper lying conditions. However, the light does not need to reach the target cells to have the treatment effect.

The most popularly described treatment benefit of LLLT is wound healing. The purpose of using LLLT as part of postoperative therapy is to provide patients with the highest quality of health care. This should include minimal discomfort or pain and a shortened healing period. It can be applied to many dental procedures, such as operative dentistry, fixed prosthetics, nonsurgical and surgical endodontic procedures, nonsurgical and surgical periodontal treatments, implantology, oral surgery, or orthodontic adjustments. Approximately 2 J of energy are applied from the wand-like probe to the patient's injection and operative sites, apical to the tooth apex buccally and lingually, around the CEJ and masticatory muscles.

The use of LLLT helps to control the symptoms and condition of periodontitis. The anti-inflammatory effect slows or stops the deterioration of periodontal tissues and reduces the swelling to facilitate the hygiene in conjunction with other scaling, root planning, curettage, or surgical treatment. As a result, there is an accelerated healing and less post-op discomfort. Studies report stimulation of human periodontal fibroblasts, reduced gingivitis index, pocket depth, plaque index, gingival fluid, and metalloproteinase-8 levels, and there are positive results after gingivectomies.

FUTURE APPLICATIONS

Although there is an extensive literature on the effects of both carbon dioxide and Nd:YAG lasers on the dental hard tissues, this area is still in a state of flux. In addition to their surgical applications, studies have indicated that lasers may be used to detect caries, measure blood flow, and assess tooth mobility. These are exciting areas of research that may prove to have substantial diagnostic benefits.

Recently, as a novel application of laser, the use of diode laser fluorescence spectroscopy for detection of dental calculus has been suggested by **Hibst et al**[38] (Diagnodent, KaVo, Biberach, Germany), which uses laser fluorescence induced by the 655 nm InGaAsP diode laser for detection of calculus that includes a significant amount of bacteria or their byproducts. It was suggested that bacteria or their byproducts might be the source of reaction to the increasing fluorescence. Hibst et al[38] identified the source of red excited fluorescence present in calculus as porphyrins, especially proto-porphyrin IX, which are products of oral bacteria, such as Prevotella intermedia and P. gingivalis.

Keller et al[46] reported a novel method of subgingival root planing with the Er:YAG laser combined with diode laser fluorescence spectroscopy. Traditionally, calculus detection has been performed manually by judging the ruggedness of the root surface using a periodontal probe. The laser fluorescence probe may be a novel, valuable tool for clinical detection of calculus in the near future. Er:YAG laser treatment combined with an automatic calculus- detecting system may be a novel technical modality for pocket therapy in the near future.

Yukna et al[90] have reported that LANAP- Laser Assisted New Attachment Procedure (using PerioLase MVP-7 from Biolase Corp.) has resulted in cementum mediated periodontal ligament new attachment to the root surface in the absence of long junctional epithelium.

Walsh et al[85] in 2003 have reported that LLP- Laser Lethal Photosensitization with photosensitizing dyes has an effective anti-microbial action against various cariogenic and periodontopathic organisms.

The **future of Laser Perio-therapy** rests on the development of newer laser systems as well as improvement of currently available laser systems, such as miniaturization of device sizes for accessibility into periodontal pockets, space-limited due to the complex root morphology and furcated roots and also advances in parameters of performance suitable for periodontal treatment. The high financial cost of the laser apparatus is still somewhat prohibitory, and this has prevented the spread of laser treatment among general practitioners. However, the price is expected to decrease with developments in laser technology and with increasing demand. Further research on the potential use of laser energy in periodontal therapy is indicated, and the scientific literature should be followed for future developments. This is an exciting field with many promising possibilities to be investigated, and represents an area that may ultimately prove to be rich with utility in the practice of Periodontics.

BIBLIOGRAPHY

1. Adrian JC: Pulp effects of neodymium laser. Oral Surgery, 301-305, August 1977.

2. Akira Miyazaki et al. Effects of Nd:YAG and CO_2 Laser Treatment and Ultrasonic Scaling on Periodontal Pockets of Chronic Periodontitis Patents. J. Periodontol 2003;74:175-180.

3. Albert Mehl, Reinhardt Wickel et al. Anti-microbial effects of Er; YAG Laser irradiation or root surfaces. J Clin Perio 2000;29:7-144-167.

4. Ando Y, Aoki A, Watanabe H, Ishikawa I. Bactericidal effect of erbium YAG laser on periodontopathic bacteria. Lasers Surg Med 1996: 19: 190–200.

5. Aoki A, Ishikawa I, Yamada T, Otsuki M, Watanabe H, Tagami J, Ando Y, Yamamoto H. Comparison between Er:YAG laser and conventional technique for root caries treatment in vitro. J Dent Res 1998: 77: 1404–1414.

6. Bach G et al. Conventional versus laser assisted therapy of peri-implantitis: a a five year comparative study. Implant Dent 2000;9(3):247-51.

7. Bader H. Use of Lasers in Periodontics. Dent. Clin North Am. 2000; 44: 779-792.

8. Barone A, Covani U, Crepsi R, Romanos GE. Root surface morphological changes after focused versus defocused carbon dioxide laser Irradiation: a scanning electron microscopy analysis. J Periodontol 2002: 73: 370–373.

9. Baxter G et al. Therapeutic lasers, Theory & practice, 1994.

10. Bauerle D (ed). Laser processing and diagnostics. Proceeding of an international conference, university of Linz,Austria,1994.

11. Burkes JE et al: Wet versus dry enamel ablation by Er.YAG laser. The journal of prosthetic dentistry,67,6, 847-851,1992.

12. Coffelt DW, Cobb CM, MacNeill S, Rapley JW, Killoy WJ. Determination of energy density threshold for laser ablation of bacteria. An in vitro study. J Clin Periodontol 1997: 24: 1–7.

13. Coleton Stuart. Lasers in surgical periodontics and oral medicine. Dent. Clin N. Am. 48(2004) 937-962.

14. Colver GB. & Priestly GC :Failure of a helium neon laser to affect components of wound healing in vitro .British journal of dermatology ,121, 179-186, 1989.

15. Colvard M & Kuo P: Managing Aphthous Ulcers: Laser treatment applied. Jada, 122, 51-53, 1991.

16. Colluzi DJ. Fundamentals of dental lasers: science and instruments. Dent Clin N Am. 48(2004) 751-770.

17. Colluzi DJ et al. Lasers and soft tissue curettage: An update compedium. 2002:23:1104-1111.

18. Colluzi DJ & Convissor RA: Atlas of laser applications in dentistry, Quintessence International, 2007.

19. Convissor RA. The biologic rationale for the use of lasers in dentistry. Dent Clin N Am. 48(2004) 771-794.

20. Convissor RA: Lasers in general dentistry; Oral & Maxillofacial clinics of North America, 16, 165-179, 2004.

21. Costello BJ: Lasers in oral & maxillofacial surgery; Anaesthesia/Dentoalveolar surgery/office management,1,372-404,2003

22. Cozean C et al: Dentistry for the 21st century, Erbium:YAG laser for the teeth. Jada,128, 1080-1097,1997.

23. Crespi R, Barone A, Covani U, Ciaglia RN, Romanos GE. Effects of carbon dioxide laser treatment on fibroblast attachment to Lasers in non surgical periodontal therapy root surfaces. A scanning electron microscopy analysis. J Periodontol 2002: 73: 1308–1312.

24. Dortbudak O et al. Lethal photosensitisation for decontamination of implant surfaces in the treatment of peri-implantitis. Oral Implants Res.2001;12(2):104-8.

25. Elsson LM : Practical laser safety in oral & maxillofacial surgery. Lasers in maxillofacial surgery and dentistry,11-16,2004.

26. Emshoff R et al : Low level laser therapy for treatment of Temporomandibular joint pain :a double blind and placebo controlled trial. "OOOOE",105,452-256,2008

27. Esen E et al: gingival melanin pigmentation and its treatment with the carbon dioxide laser, 98,5, 522-527,2004.

28. Finkbeiner RL. The results of 1328 periodontal pockets treated with the argon laser: selective pocket thermolysis. J Clin Laser Med Surg 1995: 13: 273–281.

29. Fisher SE & Frame JW : The effects of the Carbon Dioxide surgical laser on oral tissues. British journal of oral & maxillofacial surgery,22,414-425,1984.

30. Frentzen M & Koort HJ: Lasers in dentistry: new possibilities with advancing laser technology?IDJ,40,1990,323-332.

31. Fuller TA : Physical considerations of lasers; Lasers In Maxillofacial Surgery & Dentistry, 1-4,2004.

32. Gao XL et al : Laser-fluoride effect on root demineralization; TOF-SIMS,2006.

33. Gordon TE : Single surface cutting of normal tooth with ruby laser; JADA,74,398-402,1967.

34. Granados. FJA et al. Carbon Dioxide laser vermillectomy for Actnic chelitis; Oral Maxillofacial Surg, 51, 118-121,1993.

35. Gutknecht N, Gelsky H, Zimmermann R, Lampert F. Lasers in periodonology: state of the art. J Oral Laser Appl 2001: 1:169–179.

36. Guttenberg SA. Laser Physics and tissue interaction. Oral & Maxillofacial clinics of North America,16,143-147,2004.

37. Haim T et al. Gingival Depigmentation by erbium : YAG laser : clinical observations and patient responses. J. Periodontal 2003;74;1660-1667.

38. Hibst R, Paulus R, Lussi A. Detection of occlusal caries by laser fluorescence: basic and clinical investigations. Med Laser Appl 2001: 16: 205–213.

39. Horton JE, Lin PP-Y. A comparison of the Nd:YAG laser used subgingivally with root planning. The third international congress on lasers in Dentistry.Salt Lake city, University of Utah.1992; 23.

40. Israel M et al. Use of the carbon dioxide laser in retarding epithelial migration: A pilot histologic human study utilizing case reports. J. Periodontol 1995; 66: 197-204.

41. Ito K, et al. Effects of Nd. YAG laser radiation on removal of a root surface smear layer after root planning: a scanning electron microscopic study. J Periodontol 1993;64:547-52.

42. Jayawardena J.A. et al. Pulpal response to exposure with ER:YAG laser, "OOOE"91,2. 222-228,2001.

43. Jurg Ebehard et al. Efficacy of subgingival calculus removal with Er:YAG laser compared to mechanical debridement : an in situ study. J. Clin Periodontol 2003; 30; 511-518.

44. Kana.J.S et al: Effect of low power density laser radiation on healing of open skin wounds in rats. Arch Surg; 116, March 1981.

45. Kato T et al. Bactericidal efficacy of carbon dioxide laser against bacteria-contaminated titanium implant and subsequent cellular adhesion to irradiated area. Lasers Surg. Med 1998; 23(5): 299-309.

46. Keller U, Hibst R. Experimental studies of the application of the Er:YAG laser on dental hard substances. II. Light microscopic and SEM investigations. Lasers Surg Med 1989: 9: 345–351.

47. Kimura. Y et al: root surface temperature increases during Er: YAG laser irradiation of root canals. Journal of endodontics, 28, 2, 76-79, 2002.

48. Kreisler M et al. Effect of Nd:YAG, Ho:YAG, Er:YAG, carbon dioxide and GaAIAs laser irradiation on surface properties of endosseous dental implants. Int J Oral Maxillofac Implants 2002;17(2):202-11.

49. Liu CM, Shyu YC, Pei SC, Lan WH, Hou LT. In vitro effectof laser irradiation on cemen·um-bound endotoxin isolatedfrom periodontally diseased roots. J Periodontol 2002:73: 1260–12€6.

50. Martin Emile et al. Lasers in dental implantology. Dent. Clin N Am. 48(2004)999-1015.

51. Mehta J et al. Short term assessment of the Nd:YAG laser with and without sodium fluoride varnish in the treatment of dentin hypersensitivity: A clinical and scanning electron microscopic study. J. Periodontol 2005;76:1140-1147.

52. Merchant.N : Lasers in conservative dentistry and endodontics ; IDRR,

   25-26, 2007

53. Miserendino. L.J: History & Development of laser dentistry; Lasers in dentistry.

54. Miyazaki H et al : Intra-lesional laser treatment of voluminous vascular lesions in the oral cavity; "OOOOE",107,164-172,2009

55. Moritz A, Gutknecht N, Doertbudak O, Goharkhay K, Schoop U, Schauer P, Sperr W. Bacterial reduction in periodontal pockets through irradiation with a diode laser: a pilot study. J Clin Laser Med Surg 1997: 15: 33–37.

56. Moritz A, Shapiro S, Schoop U, Goharkhay K, Schauer P, Doert Budak O, Wernisch J, Sperr W. Treatment of periodontal pockets with a diode laser. Lasers Surg Med 1998: 22: 302–311.

57. Morlock BJ et al. The effect of Nd:YAG laser exposure on root surfaces when used as an adjunct to root planning : an in-vitro study. J Periodontol 1992;63:637-41

58. Mouhyi et al. Re-establishment of the atomic composition and the oxide structure of contaminated titanium surfaces by means of carbon dioxide laser and hydrogen peroxide: an in-vitro study. Clin Implant Dent Relat Res 2000; 2(4):190-202.

59. Mouhyi et al. Temperature increases during surface decontamination of titanium implants using carbon dioxide laser. Clin Oral Implants Res 1999;10(1):54-61.

60. Neill ME, Mellonig JT. Clinical efficacy of the Nd. YAG laser for combination periodontitis therapy. Pract Periodont Aesthet Dent 1997;9(6 Suppl):1-5.

61. Piccione .P.J : Dental Laser Safety; Dental clinics of North America,48,4,   795-808,2004

62. Pick MR : The use of laser for treatment of gingival diseases : "Oral & Maxillofacial clinics of North America";9,1,1-20,1997

63. Pick MR et al : The laser gingivectomy: The use of carbon dioxide laser for the removal of phenytoin hyperplasia; J Periodontology,56,8,1985

64. Rodrigues LK et al: In situ mineral loss inhibition by carbon dioxide laser and fluoride; journal of dental research,85,7,617-621,2000.

65. Romanos et al. Laser surgical tools in implant dentistry for the long term diagnosis of each implant. Int. Cong. Ser2004;1248:112-3.

66. Rossmann J. Lasers in periodontics. J. Periodontol 2002; 73: 1231-9.

67. Rossmann J et al. Retardation of epithelial migration in monkeys using a carbon dioxide laser. An animal study. J Periodontol 1992; 63: 902-907.

68. Schwarz F et al. Influence of an Er:YAG laser on the surface structure of titanium implants. Schweiz Montasschr Zahnmed 2003;113(6):660-71.

69. Schwarz F et al. In vivo and in vitro effects of an Er:YAG laser, a GaAlAs diode laser, and scaling and root planing on periodontally diseased root surfaces : a comparative histologic study. Lasers Surg Med 2003; 32: 359-66.

70. Schwarz F, Putz N, Georg T, Reich E. Effect of an Er:YAG laser on periodontally involved root surfaces: an in vivo and in vitro SEM comparison. Lasers Surg Med 2001: 29:328–335.

71. Sculean A, Araujo H, Schwarz F, Berakdar M, Arweiler N, Becker J.Periodontal treatment with an Er:YAG laser compared to ultrasonic instrumentation. J Periodontol 2004: 75: 974–981.

72. Seka W, Featherstone JDB, Fried D, Visuri SR, Walsh JT. Laser ablation of dental hard tissue: from explosive ablation to plasma-mediated ablation. Proc SPIE 1996: 2672: 144–158.

73. Sexton J & O'Hare D :Simplified treatment of vascular lesions using the Argon laser; J Oral Maxillofacial Surg,51,12-16,1993

74. Smith PW: The soft laser: Therapeutic tool or popular placebo?; "OOO",66,654-658,1988

75. Spencer P et al. Chemical characterization of lased root surfaces using fourier transform infrared photoacoustic spectroscopy. J Periodontol 1992;63:633-6.

76. Strang R & Carmichael A: Soft Lasers-have they a place in dentistry?BDJ,24,221-225,1988

77. Strauss RA et al. Lasers in contemporary oral & maxillofacial surgery. Dent Clin N Am. 48(2004)861-888.

78. Sun Grace et al. Low level laser therapy in dentistry. Dent Clin N Am. 48(2004) 1061-1076.

79. Tewfik HM, et al. Structural and functional changes of cementum surface following exposure to a modified Nd. YAG laser. J Periodontol 1994;65:297-302.

80. Thomas D. et al. Effects of the Nd. YAG laser and combined treatments on in-vitro fibroblast attachment to root surfaces. J Periodontol 2000:1994:21:38-44.

81. Trylovich D et al. The effect of the Nd. YAG laser on in-vitro fibroblast attachment to endotoxin treated root surfaces. J Periodontol 200;1992(63):626-32.

82. Tucker D, Cobb CM, Rapley JW, Killoy WJ. Morphologic changes following in vitro carbon dioxide laser treatment of calculus-laden root surfaces. Lasers Surg Med 1996: 18:150–156.

83. Watanabe H, Ishikawa I, Suzuki M, Hasegawa K. Clinical assessments of the erbium:YAG laser for soft tissue surgery and scaling. J Clin Laser Med Surg 1996: 14: 67–75.

84. Walsh LJ, Flotte TJ, Deutsch TF. Er:YAG laser ablation of tissue: effect of pulse duration and tissue type on thermal damage. Lasers Surg Med 1989: 9: 314–326.

85. Walsh LJ: The current status of laser application in dentistry. Australian dental journal, 143- 154, 2003.

86. Wheeland RG : Cosmetic use of lasers; Cosmetic Dermatology, 13,2,447-459, 1995.

87. White JM et al: Effects of pulsed Nd:YAG laser energy on human teeth; Three year follow up study. JADA, 124, 45-51, 1993.

88. White JM, Goodis HE, Yessik MJ, Myers TD. Histologic effects of a high-repetition pulsed Nd:YAG laser on intra oral soft tissue. Proc SPIE 1995: 2394: 143–153.

89. Yamaguchi H, Kobayashi K, Osada R, Sakuraba E, Nomura T, Arai T, Nakamura J. Effects of irradiation of an erbium: YAG laser on root surfaces. J Periodontol 1997: 68: 1151– 1155.

90. Yukna RA, Evans GH, Vastardis S, Carr RF. Human periodontal regeneration following the laser assisted new attachment procedure. Int Assoc Dent Res 2004; 52:396-403.

91. Zharikov EV et al. Stimulated emission from Er3+ ions in yttrium alminum garnet crystals at k ¼ 2.94l. SovJ Quantum Electron 1975: 4: 1039–1040.

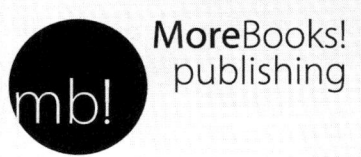
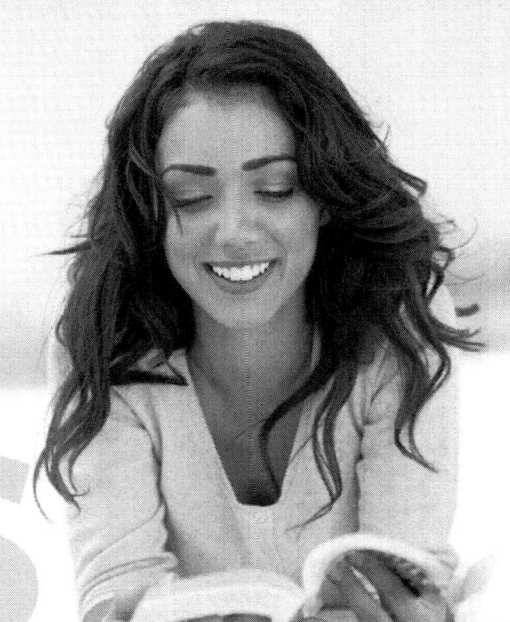
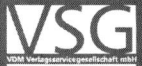

Printed in Great Britain
by Amazon.co.uk, Ltd.,
Marston Gate.